acupressure

how to cure common ailments the natural way

Michael Reed Gach PhD

piatkus

To my grandmother
who expressed to me as a little boy
the greatest unconditional love through her hands, eyes, and heart.

The depth and power of our affectionate exchange
still fills me with the determination to enhance other lives
by teaching the ancient art of hands-on healing.

ACKNOWLEDGMENTS

I am grateful for the love I have received from my parents, teachers, and friends. I especially want to thank my students, clients, staff, and the faculty at the Acupressure Institute — my extended family and community for over fifteen years — for the professional support I needed to write this book.

I want to acknowledge all my teachers but particularly Iona and Ron Teeguarden and Frank Chung, C.A., O.M.D., who taught me the practical therapeutic applications of acupressure's potent points.

The guidance and strong editorial contributions from Sally Zahner and Leslie Meredith transformed my manuscript into a comprehensive whole. I appreciate their insight, talents, and the tremendous amount of work they gave my book. I also want to thank Gina Velasquez for handling everything from editorial details to coordinating production.

I want to thank Paul Abell, Ph.D., Pamela Clarke, Joseph Carter, C.A., Alice Hiatt, R.N., and Brian O'Dea, C.A., for their technical advice and suggestions. I am especially grateful for the help of Cathy Hemming and Patty Leasure in getting this book published.

In terms of producing the way the book looks, Mary Sanichas, with her high-tech scanner and fully computerized desktop publishing expertise, did an outstanding job with the book's graphic design. I am also grateful for the organizational and editorial computer work of Carrie Sealine.

I enjoyed working with David Lehrer again, who shot all of the fine photography in this book. Joan Carol, Christel Busch, and Gordon Pagnello certainly deserve acknowledgment for their anatomical drawings.

Finally, I want to express my appreciation to the models in the book: Molly Beck, Joella Caskey, Pamela Clarke, Nathan Hiatt, Herb R. Jorgensen, Alexander B. Levin, Takami Matsumoto, Bill Mathers, Frank Nuessle, Gene Poferl, Mary Sanichas, and Jo Ann Turner.

TABLE OF CONTENTS

PREFACE

This book presents in easy steps how you can use acupressure on yourself to relieve stress-related problems, both physical and emotional. These potent points and self-care exercises will enable you to participate actively in your own healing. At the same time, however, you should continue to see your doctor for individualized examinations, advice, and treatment. I believe that this book can complement your medical care by enabling you to take a vital role in getting and staying well.

This book is not intended as a substitute for medical advice of physicians. The reader should regularly consult a physician in matters relating to his or her health and particularly in respect to any symptoms that may require diagnosis or medical attention. Before utilizing acupressure, the reader should be certain to read all of Part I and the entire chapter relating to the ailment and to observe any specific cautions given in the book. Pregnant women should be certain to read Chapter 36.

Part I gives you general information about acupressure, its origins, how it works, what it is good and not good for, what a point is, how to find the points, and how to apply finger pressure. Part II contains forty chapters of fully illustrated self-care methods for relieving common complaints from acne to headaches to wrist pain.

The ailments I deal with are organized alphabetically to enable you to find your problem easily. First, I discuss each complaint, giving some of its causes and tips for prevention. Then specific acupressure points that can relieve the symptoms are shown in illustrations, so that you can find them easily. I then present step-by-step routines for using acupressure and end each chapter with a list of other chapters that contain additional points for further relief. The index further guides you to find the potent points for relieving other problems.

It is a tremendous blessing to be able to help yourself and others, without costly equipment, simply using your hands, at any time, wherever you are. I hope that this book will lead you to a new dimension of well-being — not only to be able to work actively to improve your health, but to expand your awareness of your own healing energy and potent life spirit.

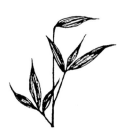

Part I

INTRODUCTION TO ACUPRESSURE

Its Origins, Uses, and Guidelines

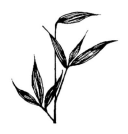

PIATKUS

First published in Great Britain in 1992 by Piatkus Books
This paperback edition published in 2004 by Piatkus

9 11 13 15 17 19 20 18 16 14 12 10

A CIP catalogue record for this book
is available from the British Library.

ISBN 978-0-7499-2534-5

Printed and bound by CPI Group (UK) Ltd, Croydon, CR0 4YY

Papers used by Piatkus are from well-managed forests
and other responsible sources.

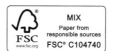

Piatkus
An imprint of
Little, Brown Book Group
Carmelite House
50 Victoria Embankment
London EC4Y 0DZ

An Hachette UK Company
www.hachette.co.uk

www.improvementzone.co.uk

Important Note:
This book is not intended as a substitute for medical advice or treatment.
Any person with a condition requiring medical attention should
consult a qualified medical practitioner or suitable therapist.

1
WHAT IS ACUPRESSURE?

Acupressure is an ancient healing art that uses the fingers to press key points on the surface of the skin to stimulate the body's natural self-curative abilities. When these points are pressed, they release muscular tension and promote the circulation of blood and the body's life force to aid healing. Acupuncture and acupressure use the same points, but acupuncture employs needles, while acupressure uses the gentle but firm pressure of hands (and even feet). There is a massive amount of scientific data that demonstrates why and how acupuncture is effective. But acupressure, the older of the two traditions, was neglected after the Chinese developed more technological methods for stimulating points with needles and electricity. Acupressure, however, continues to be the most effective method for self-treatment of tension-related ailments by using the power and sensitivity of the human hand.

Foremost among the advantages of acupressure's healing touch is that it is safe to do on yourself and others — even if you've never done it before — so long as you follow the instructions and pay attention to the cautions. There are no side effects from drugs, because there are no drugs. And the only equipment needed are your own two hands. You can practice acupressure therapy any time, anywhere.

My clinical experiences over the past eighteen years have shown me that acupressure can be effective in helping relieve headaches, eyestrain, sinus problems, neck pain, backaches, arthritis, muscle aches, and tension due to stress. I have also shown hundreds of my acupressure students, patients, and friends how to use acupressure to relieve ulcer pain,

menstrual cramps, lower back aches, constipation, and indigestion. You can also use self-acupressure to relieve anxiety and to help you get to sleep at night.

Susan, a student of mine, was suffering from insomnia and occasional headaches for many years, as the result of a neck injury. "I feel so tired and weary, nearly all the time, Michael," she said. "Can acupressure points help me?"

I showed her several potent points on her ankles and neck for headaches, as well as some upper-back stretching exercises for her insomnia. Susan reported to me two weeks later, glowing. "The treatment really worked! I've been sleeping uninterrupted and soundly through the night for the first time in fifteen years."

There are also great advantages to using acupressure as a way to balance the body and maintain good health. The healing touch of acupressure reduces tension, increases circulation, and enables the body to relax deeply. By relieving stress, acupressure strengthens resistance to disease and promotes wellness.

In acupressure, local symptoms are considered an expression of the condition of the body as a whole. A tension headache, for instance, may be rooted in the shoulder and neck area. Thus acupressure focuses on relieving pain and discomfort as well as on responding to tension before it develops into a "dis-ease," that is, before the constrictions and imbalances can do further damage. By using a combination of self-help methods such as trigger point stimulation, deep breathing, range-of-motion exercises, and relaxation techniques, you can improve your condition as well as feel more alive, healthy, and in harmony with your life.

Recently, Judy, one of my advanced acupressure students, complained about having night sweats. She was in the midst of making a serious decision about where to live, which also involved a relationship that was troubling her. I immediately noticed that her upper back was rounded by tension and discovered even more tension in her neck. I showed her the points for working on these areas. A month later, after using acupressure on herself twice a day, Judy reported that much of her upper back tension and a "ball" of deep anxiety had dissipated. She also felt clearer and more objective in dealing with her problems. Best of all, the night sweats that had made her miserable for two months were gone.

Alice, one of my elderly clients, had limited mobility in her neck with severe arthritic neck pain that radiated down her shoulders into her arms as well as up into her head. After her first acupressure session, she not only felt less discomfort but also had greater flexibility in her neck. For the first time in years, she was able to move her head freely without pain.

After several weeks Alice realized that she could help herself using the points underneath the base of her skull to relieve both her neck pain and stiffness. Recently she told me that whenever the pain "creeps up on her," she practices self-acupressure. It is possible that this increased mobility, in turn, prevents further deterioration.

The Development of Acupressure

The origins of acupressure are as ancient as the instinctive impulse to hold your forehead or temples when you have a headache. Everyone at one time or another has used his or her hands spontaneously to hold tense or painful places on the body.

More than 5,000 years ago, the Chinese discovered that pressing certain points on the body relieved pain where it occurred and also benefited other parts of the body more remote from the pain and the pressure point.[1] Gradually, they found other locations that not only alleviated pain but also influenced the functioning of certain internal organs.

In the early Chinese dynasties, when stones and arrows were the only implements of war, many soldiers wounded on the battlefield reported that symptoms of disease that had plagued them for years had suddenly vanished. Naturally, such strange occurrences baffled the physicians who could find no logical relationship between the trauma and the ensuing recovery of health. After years of meticulous observation, ancient Chinese physicians developed ways of curing certain illnesses by striking or piercing specific points on the surface of the body.[2]

As with the Chinese soldiers, people through the ages have found the most effective ways to help themselves by trial and error. The art and science of acupressure was practiced by the contributions of people whose awareness was so highly developed that they could feel where the bodies of people in pain were constricted and sense which trigger points would alleviate the problem. The Chinese have practiced self-acupressure for over 5,000 years as a way of keeping themselves well and happy. You, too, can learn how to complement the care you receive from your doctors. You can help your body relieve itself of common ailments, such as those in this book, by pressing the proper spots, which I will teach you. In the course of trying out these points, you may even find others that work better for you.

Many of the health problems in our society — from bad backs to arthritis — are the result of living unnaturally. Stress, tension, lack of exercise, poor eating habits, and poor posture contribute to the epidemic of

---

[1] Ilza Veith, trans., *The Yellow Emperor's Classic of Internal Medicine* (Berkeley: University of California Press, 1949). An ancient Chinese medical text.
[2] Dr. Stephen Thomas Chang, *The Complete Book of Acupuncture* (Berkeley: Celestial Arts, 1976), 14.

degenerative diseases in our culture. Acupressure is one way to help your body fight back and balance itself in the face of the pressures of modern life.

How Acupressure Works

Acupressure points (also called potent points) are places on the skin that are especially sensitive to bioelectrical impulses in the body and conduct those impulses readily. Traditionally, Asian cultures conceived of the points as junctures of special pathways that carried the human energy that the Chinese call *chi* and the Japanese call *ki*. Western scientists have also mapped out and proven the existence of this system of body points by using sensitive electrical devices.

Stimulating these points with pressure, needles, or heat triggers the release of *endorphins*, which are the neurochemicals that relieve pain. As a result, pain is blocked and the flow of blood and oxygen to the affected area is increased. This causes the muscles to relax and promotes healing.

Because acupressure inhibits the pain signals sent to the brain through a mild, fairly painless stimulation, it has been described as closing the "gates" of the pain-signaling system, preventing painful sensations from passing through the spinal cord to the brain.[3]

Besides relieving pain, acupressure can help rebalance the body by dissolving tensions and stresses that keep it from functioning smoothly and that inhibit the immune system. Acupressure enables the body to adapt to environmental changes and resist illness.

Tension tends to concentrate around acupressure points. When a muscle is chronically tense or in spasm, the muscle fibers contract due to the secretion of lactic acid caused by fatigue, trauma, stress, chemical imbalances, or poor circulation. For instance,

when you are under a great deal of stress you may find you have difficulty breathing. Certain acupressure points relieve chest tension and enable you to breathe deeply.

As a point is pressed, the muscle tension yields to the finger pressure, enabling the fibers to elongate and relax, blood to flow freely, and toxins to be released and eliminated. Increased circulation also brings more oxygen and other nutrients to affected areas. This increases the body's resistance to illness and promotes a longer, healthier, more vital life. When the blood and bioelectrical energy circulate properly, we have a greater sense of harmony, health, and well-being.

Ways to Use Acupressure

Acupressure's potent points can be used to enhance many aspects of life. In addition to managing stress, you can use acupressure to relieve and prevent sports injuries. Sports massage has been widely used by athletes before and after Olympic events. Acupressure complements sports medicine treatments by using points and massage techniques to improve muscle tone and circulation and relieve neuromuscular problems.

The Chinese have also used acupressure as a beauty treatment for thousands of years. You can use potent points to improve skin condition and tone and relax the facial muscles, which can lessen the appearance of wrinkles without drugs.

Although acupressure is not a substitute for medical care, it is often an appropriate complementary treatment. It can, for instance, speed the healing of a broken bone once it has been set, or aid a cancer patient by helping to alleviate some of the associated pain and anxiety of the disease.

Similarly, acupressure can be an effective adjunct to chiropractic treatment. By relaxing and toning the back muscles, acupressure makes the spinal adjustments easier and more effective, and the results last longer. In fact, the two therapies were originally practiced together in ancient China.

[3] T. Tan Leng, Margaret Y. C. Tan, and Ilza Veith, *Acupuncture Therapy — Current Chinese Practice* (Philadelphia: Temple University, 1973).

Psychotherapy patients can derive benefits from acupressure by using it to heighten body awareness and deal with stress. When powerful emotions are free and unresolved, the body stores the resulting tension in the muscles. Acupressure can help restore emotional balance by releasing the accumulated tension caused by repressed feelings.

An acupressure point actually has two identities and ways of working. When you stimulate a point in the same area where you feel pain or tension, it's called a *local* point. That same point can also relieve pain in a part of the body that is distant from the point, in which case it is called a *trigger* point. This triggering mechanism works through a human electrical channel called a *meridian*. The meridians are pathways that connect the acupressure points to each other as well as to the internal organs. Just as blood vessels carry the blood that nourishes the body physically, the meridians are distinct channels that circulate electrical energy throughout the body. They are thought to be part of a master communications system of universal life energy, connecting the organs with all sensory, physiological, and emotional aspects of the body. This physical network of energy also contains key points that we can use to deepen our spiritual awareness as we heal ourselves.

Because the stimulation of one point can send a healing message to other parts of the body, each acupressure point can benefit a variety of complaints and symptoms. Therefore, in the following chapters you will find a particular acupressure point used for a variety of problems. The highly effective acupressure point in the webbing between your thumb and index finger,[4] for instance, is not only beneficial for relieving arthritic pain in the hand, but also benefits the colon and relieves problems in the facial area and the head, including headaches, toothaches, and sinus problems.

Tonic points[5] improve your condition and maintain general health. They strengthen the overall body system and fortify various internal organs and vital systems of the body.

How to Find a Point: Acupressure Point Names and Reference Numbers

You locate an acupressure point by referring to anatomical landmarks. To help you find them, all of the points in this book are illustrated with a description of these landmarks (such as bone indentations and protrusions).

Some acupressure points lie underneath major muscle groups. While points located near a bone structure usually lie in an indentation, muscular points lie within a muscular cord, band, or knot of tension. To stimulate the point, press directly on the cord or into the hollow.

As acupressure evolved, each of the 365 points was named poetically, originally with a Chinese character. The imagery of its name offers insight into either a point's benefits or location. For instance, the name Hidden Clarity refers to the mental benefit of the point: It clears the mind. Shoulder's Corner refers to that point's location. The Three Mile Point earned its name because it gives a person an extra three miles of energy. Runners and hikers have used this famous point to increase stamina and endurance.

Some of the names of the acupressure points also serve as a powerful meditation tool. By pressing a point and silently repeating its name while you visualize its benefit and breathe deeply, you can realize the full potential power that each point offers. As you hold the Sea of Vitality points in your lower back, breathe deeply and visualize each breath replenishing your deep reservoir of vitality. Use the power of your mind to strengthen and help heal your lower back.

---

[4] **Caution:** This point is forbidden during pregnancy, because its stimulation can cause premature contractions in the uterus.

[5] For additional information on tonic points, see Michael Reed Gach, *Greater Energy at Your Fingertips* (Berkeley: Celestial Arts, 1986), 9-25.

You can create affirmations with the names of the points — powerful action statements that amplify a point's benefits. For example, hold the Letting Go points on the upper, outer chest with your fingertips. Breathe deeply. Imagine yourself letting go of tension, frustration, and stress. As you hold and breathe into these points, repeat to yourself that you are now letting go of all negativity and irritability.

In addition to its name, each point was assigned an identification number to track its placement along the body. Point location numbers, such as St 3 or GB 21, are a standard referencing system used by professional acupressurists and acupuncturists and so I use them as an additional label, too. These notations are explained in the Glossary, but you do not need to know or remember any of these numbers to practice the self-acupressure techniques in this book.

The Third Eye:
A Potent Spiritual Point

Using the healing touch of acupressure can also be a practical way of deepening your spiritual life. By lightly touching the Third Eye Point, for instance, just above the bridge of the nose, for a couple of minutes, you can enhance your inner awareness. If you want to progress further, meditate on this point for five to ten minutes each day, and within a few weeks, you may notice that your intuition will begin to increase. Concentrating on the Third Eye Point can nourish your spiritual nature.

Spirituality is not disembodied; the most powerful spiritual experiences are rooted in one's body. When I close my eyes and lightly touch the Third Eye Point, and completely focus my attention on that spot between my eyebrows, I heighten my sense of myself. I become intensely aware of how my body feels, how my breathing feels. As I sense the blood pulsing throughout my body, I experience the flow of life energy. And if I continue breathing deeply, sitting with my spine straight, I become aware of every part of my body at once — as a harmonious, unified presence. When I meditate, this often leads to a powerful sense of oneness with the world. Acupressure's potent power can heal us both physically and spiritually.

The healing benefits of acupressure involve both the relaxation of the body and its positive effects on the mind. As tension is released, you not only feel good physically, but you also feel better emotionally and mentally. When your body relaxes, your mind relaxes as well, creating another state of consciousness. This expanded awareness leads to mental clarity and a healthier physical and emotional healing, dissolving the division between the mind and body.

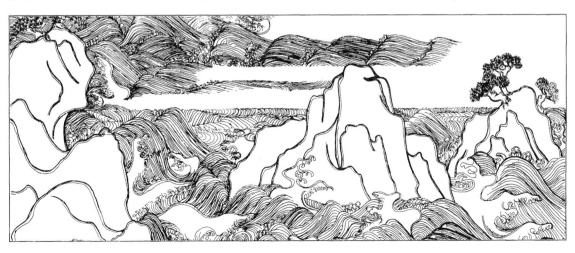

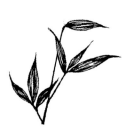

2
PRACTICING SELF-ACUPRESSURE

Several different kinds of acupressure are currently practiced, although the same ancient trigger points are used in all of them. Varying rhythms, pressures, and techniques create different styles of acupressure, just as different forms of music use the same notes but combine them in distinctive ways. Shiatsu, for instance, the most well-known style of acupressure, can be quite vigorous, with firm pressure applied to each point for only three to five seconds. Another kind of acupressure gently holds each point for a minute or more. Pressing with an intermittent, fast beat is stimulating; a slower pressure creates a deeply relaxing effect on the body.

Acupressure Massage Techniques

We'll use the following techniques in the exercises throughout the book.

Firm pressure is the most fundamental technique. Use thumbs, fingers, palms, the side of the hand, or knuckles to apply steady, stationary pressure. To relax an area or relieve pain, apply pressure gradually and hold without any movement for several minutes at a time. One minute of steady pressure (when applied gradually) calms and relaxes the nervous system, promoting greater healing. To stimulate the area, apply pressure for only four or five seconds.

Slow motion kneading uses the thumbs and fingers along with the heels of the hands to squeeze large muscle groups firmly. The motion is similar to that of kneading a large mass of dough. Simply lean the weight of your upper body into the muscle as you press to make it soft and pliable. This relieves general stiffness, shoulder and neck tension, constipation, and spasms in the calf muscles.

Brisk rubbing uses friction to stimulate the blood and lymph. Rub the skin lightly to relieve chilling, swelling, and numbness by increasing circulation, as well as to benefit the nerves and tone of the skin.

Quick tapping with fingertips stimulates muscles on unprotected, tender areas of the body such as the face. For larger areas of the body, such as the back or buttocks, use a loose fist. This can improve the functioning of nerves and sluggish muscles in the area.

Caution: If you have a serious illness or chronic or life-threatening illness such as heart disease, cancer, or high blood pressure, you should not use the following techniques described in these exercises: brisk rubbing, deep pressure, kneading, or other recommendations that may be overstimulating.

How to Apply Pressure

Use prolonged finger pressure directly on the point; gradual, steady, penetrating pressure for approximately three minutes is ideal. Each point will feel somewhat different when you press it; some points feel tense, while others are often sore or ache when pressed. How much pressure to apply to any point depends on how fit you are. A general guideline to follow is that the pressure should be firm enough so that it "hurts good" — in other words, something between pleasant, firm pressure and outright pain. The more developed the muscles are, the more pressure you should apply. If you feel extreme (or increasing) sensitivity or pain, gradually decrease the pressure until you find a balance between pain and pleasure. Acupressure is not meant to increase your tolerance of pain, so do not think of it as a test of endurance. Do not continue to press a point that is excruciatingly painful. Usually, however, if you firmly hold the point long enough (up to 2 minutes using the middle finger with your index and ring fingers on either side as support), the pain will diminish.

Note that sometimes when you hold a point, you'll feel pain in another part of your body. This phenomenon is called referred pain and indicates that those areas are related. You should press points in these related areas as well to release blockages.

The middle finger is the longest and strongest of your fingers and is best suited for applying self-acupressure. The thumb is strong, too, but often lacks sensitivity. If you find that your hand is generally weak or hurts when you apply finger pressure, you can use the knuckles or your fist or other tools, such as an avocado pit, a golf ball, or a pencil eraser.

Although you may be tempted to massage or rub the entire area, it is best just to hold the point steadily with direct finger pressure. The rule of thumb is to apply slow, firm pressure on the point at a 90 degree angle from the surface of the skin. If you are pulling the skin, then the angle of pressure is incorrect. Consciously and gradually direct the pressure into the center of the part of the body you are working on. It's important to apply and release finger pressure gradually because this allows the tissues time to respond, promoting healing. The better your concentration as you move your fingers slowly into and out of the point, the more effective the treatment will be.

After repeated acupressure sessions using different degrees of pressure, you will begin to feel a pulse at the point. This pulsation is a good sign — it means that circulation has increased. Pay attention to the type of pulse you feel. If it's very faint or throbbing, hold the point longer until the pulse balances.

If your hand gets tired, slowly withdraw pressure from the point, gently shake out your hand, and take a few deep breaths. When you're ready, go back to the point and gradually apply pressure until you reach the depth where it hurts good. Again, press directly on the painful site (which often moves, so follow and stay with it) until you feel a clear, regular pulse or until the pain diminishes. Then slowly decrease the finger pressure, ending with about twenty seconds of light touch.

When you have located the point and your fingers are comfortably positioned right on the spot, gradually lean your weight toward the point to apply the pressure. If you're pressing a point on your foot, for instance, bend your leg and apply pressure by slowly leaning forward. Using the weight of your upper body (and not just your hands) enables you to apply firm pressure without strain. Direct the pressure perpendicularly to the surface of the skin as you take several long, slow, deep breaths. Hold for a few minutes until you feel a regular pulse or until the soreness at the point decreases. Then gradually release the pressure, finishing with a light, soothing touch.

Each body — and each area of the body — requires a different amount of pressure. If it hurts a great deal when you apply pressure on a point, then use light touch instead of pressure. The calves, the face, and genital areas are sensitive. The back, buttocks, and shoulders, especially if the musculature is developed, usually need deeper, firmer pressure. Because certain areas of the body, such as the back and shoulders, are hard to reach, I will recommend using Acu-Yoga[6] postures, which involve leaning against the floor to apply the proper amount of pressure to the points.

To achieve the full benefit of self-acupressure, you should choose a comfortable, private environment that lends itself to deep relaxation. You can use acupressure at work, however, if you can take a ten-minute break. Choose whatever position you find most comfortable — either sitting or lying down. As you press points in different areas, feel free to reposition your body so that your muscles

---

[6] For further self-help information, see Michael Reed Gach *Acu-Yoga* (Tokyo: Japan Publications, 1981), 121-247.

can relax completely. (See "Guidance for Deep Relaxation," at the beginning of Part II.)

Ideally, you should wear comfortable clothing. Tight collars, belts, pants, or shoes can obstruct circulation. I recommend wearing natural fibers that breathe, such as cotton or wool blends. Also, it's a good idea to keep your fingernails trimmed fairly short to prevent any discomfort or injury to the skin.

Avoid practicing acupressure right before a big meal or on a full stomach. Wait until at least an hour after eating a light meal and even longer after eating a heavy meal. Practicing a complete acupressure routine when your stomach is full can inhibit the flow of blood and may cause nausea. However, simply pressing one or two points to relieve indigestion or hiccups is perfectly safe. Avoid iced drinks (especially during the winter months), because extreme cold generally weakens your system and can counteract the benefits of acupressure. A cup of hot herbal tea would be good after an acupressure session along with a period of deep relaxation.

For optimal results, you should perform the acupressure routines daily, whether you are using acupressure to maintain your health or to help relieve an ailment. If you are using acupressure for the latter reason, continue using these same points even after you've obtained relief. This can prevent recurrence. If you cannot practice every day, treating yourself to acupressure two or three times a week can still be effective.

Limit your self-acupressure sessions to an hour at the most. When you begin practicing acupressure, you may find that you are most comfortable holding a point for two to three minutes. You may find that you can gradually — over two to three months — work up to holding points longer, but do not hold any one point longer than ten minutes. And do not work any single area of the body, such as the abdominal area or the face, for longer that 15 minutes. The effects of acupressure can be quite strong. If you work too long, too much energy is released and complications, such as nausea and headaches, can occur.

Deep Breathing

Breathing is the most profoundly effective tool known for purifying and revitalizing the body. When your breath is shallow, all your body's vital systems function at a minimum level. If your breath is long and deep, however, the respiratory system functions properly, and the body cells become fully oxygenated. Deep breathing helps the potent points release any pain or tension and encourages healing energy to flow throughout the body. As you practice the self-acupressure routines in this book and concentrate on breathing deeply into your abdomen, you will help your body heal itself and generate a great feeling of well-being.

Concentrated breathing can especially help you better use a potent point that is painful. Close your eyes, focus your attention on the painful spot, breathe deeply, and imagine that you are breathing healing energy into the affected area as you hold the point gently. Inhale deeply into the abdomen, letting your belly expand. Feel the breath reach into the depths of the belly. Exhale slowly, letting the energy that you drew in now circulate throughout your body. Do not use a massaging movement. Focus on breathing into the pain for three full minutes. Often, poor circulation is indicated by a point that is sore when pressed. By taking long, deep breaths and pressing gently for three minutes you will close the nervous system's pain gates and help the area heal. This breathing technique will enhance the healing benefits of all the acupressure routines in this book.

Cautions to Consider

- Apply finger pressure in a slow, rhythmic manner to enable the layers of tissue and the internal organs to respond. Never press any area in an abrupt, forceful, or jarring way.
- Use the abdominal points cautiously, especially if you are ill. Avoid the abdominal area entirely if you have a life-threatening disease, especially intestinal cancer,

tuberculosis, serious cardiac conditions, and leukemia. Avoid the abdominal area during pregnancy as well.

- Special care should be taken during pregnancy. Please refer to chapter 36 for further guidance.
- Lymph areas, such as the groin, the area of the throat just below the ears, and the outer breast near the armpits, are very sensitive. These areas should be touched only lightly and not pressed.
- Do not work directly on a serious burn, an ulcerous condition, or an infection: for these conditions, medical care alone is indicated.
- Do not work directly on a recently formed scar. During the first month after an injury or operation, do not apply pressure directly on the affected site. However, gentle continuous holding a few inches away from the periphery of the injury will stimulate the area and help it heal.
- After an acupressure session, your body heat is lowered; thus your resistance to cold is also lower. Because the tensions have been released, your body's vital energies are concentrating inward to maximize healing. Your body will be more vulnerable, so be sure to wear extra clothing and keep warm when you finish an acupressure routine.

Limitations of Acupressure

Patients with life-threatening diseases and serious medical problems should always consult their doctor before using acupressure or other alternative therapies. It is important for the novice to use caution in any medical emergency situation, such as a stroke or heart attack, or for any serious medical condition, such as arteriosclerosis or an illness caused by bacteria. Nor is acupressure an appropriate sole treatment for cancer, contagious skin diseases, or sexually transmitted diseases. In conjunction with proper medical attention, however, gentle acupressure (safely away from the diseased area and the internal organs) can help soothe and relieve a patient's distress and pain. According to Dr. Serizawa,

a Japanese physician, who regularly uses acupressure in his medical research and practice:

The ailments from which [acupressure] can offer relief are numerous and include the following: symptoms of chilling; flushing; pain, and numbness; . . . headaches; heaviness in the head; dizziness; ringing in the ears; stiff shoulders arising from disorders of the autonomic nervous system; constipation; sluggishness; chills of the hands and feet; insomnia; malformations of the backbone frequent in middle age and producing pain in the shoulders, arms, and hands; pains in the back; pains in the knees experienced during standing or going up or down stairs.[7]

The following chapters provide you with ways to help yourself cope with these and other discomforts. But before you look up the specific ailments you want to know about, take a few minutes to answer the questions on the following form.

Acupressure Diary

Acupressure's effects can be subtle and while you may often experience immediate relief from stress and pain, sometimes it may take you a few weeks to notice a big change in your overall condition. In the meantime, you can use the form to the right to record your week-by-week progress. Note your body's responses to specific points and self-help techniques. Your account of which points you use, the techniques that help you most, and the time it took to achieve results can be a valuable record for learning about your body and becoming more aware of its needs.

Keep track of the results of your self-acupressure practice to pay close attention to your progress and well-being.

---

[7] Katsusuke Serizawa, M.D., *Tsubo: Vital Points for Oriental Therapy* (Tokyo: Japan Publications, 1976), 38.

Documenting Your Acupressure Progress

I would like to relieve the following ailments:

❑ Pain in my _____

❑ Tension in my _____

❑ Numbness in my _____

❑ Skin problems on my _____

❑ Other _____

I have been practicing the self-acupressure instructions in:

Chapter Number _____, called_____, on pages ____ - _____

Chapter Number _____, called_____, on pages ____ - _____

I plan to do these exercises: ❑ 10   ❑ 20   ❑ 30   ❑ 45   ❑ 60 minutes a day

Mark the drawings to the right in red ink where you feel discomfort; mark the points you have used in blue ink.

The following conditions or situations seem to make my ailment(s) worse:

❑ Standing ❑ Cold weather
❑ Menstruation ❑ Constipation
❑ Lack of exercise ❑ Stress
❑ Traveling ❑ Other _____

Describe the changes you noticed during the first three days of doing your potent points exercises regularly:

_____

_____

_____

Describe the changes you felt after one full week of self-acupressure:

_____

_____

Describe the changes you noticed in your condition and in your overall feeling of well-being after two or three weeks of doing self-acupressure:

_____

_____

Part II

ACUPRESSURE

POINTS & TECHNIQUES

FOR SPECIFIC AILMENTS

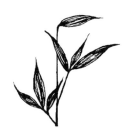

*T*he chapters in this section are organized alphabetically by symptom to make it easy for you to find the points and techniques for treating a specific ailment. Each chapter is self contained; therefore, you can skip around to explore the chapter topics you are most interested in. Use the Quick Reference Guide below to find the chapters that cover the topics related to your condition.

In each chapter, you will find an introduction to the disorder, illustrations of the acupressure points that are effective for relieving it, and step-by-step instructions on how best to apply pressure to the points. At the end of each chapter, you'll find references to other chapters that contain additional points and information related to that ailment. Also, because each acupressure point is effective for relieving many different ailments, I've listed all of the ways the point will benefit

you. So a point that I discuss in the chapter on headaches, for instance, will include a complete list of benefits even if they don't relate just to headaches.

The first few times you practice these acupressure techniques, it will naturally take you some time to master the exercises. But once you have learned the patterns, each exercise should take only ten to twenty minutes. Although the routines detailed in the following chapters are most effective if practiced in their entirety, you can still benefit from using just one or two of the points listed. I have found that the best results occur when the points are stimulated several times throughout the day. Therefore, I recommend that you do self-acupressure two or three times a day, whenever it's convenient. However, you will still derive some benefit even if you practice only a few times a week.

Quick Reference Guide

Practicing Self-Acupressure with Deep Relaxation

Ideally, these self-care exercises should be practiced in a quiet, relaxing environment to support your healing process. To begin a self-acupressure routine, I would suggest you gently stretch your body. First, reach your arms upward, as you might do when getting up in the morning. Then slowly move your torso forward, gently stretching the back of your legs, but only as far as is absolutely comfortable. Then find your most comfortable lounging chair or simply lie down on a carpeted floor.

When you finish practicing an acupressure routine from one of the proceeding chapters, follow it with the deep relaxation exercise below. Instead of rushing off to do other things, be sure to leave yourself at least five or ten minutes at the end of your acupressure session to gain the full benefits of this deeply relaxing and healing state.

The Flexibility of Self-Acupressure

You can turn a less-than-ideal environment for practicing self-acupressure, such as an airport terminal, office, or airplane, into an ideal one, with a little creativity or concentration. Headphones can provide you with a symphony of healing sounds and you can imagine yourself in a relaxed environment at home or on a quiet beach, listening to the healing sounds of the waves. Most self-acupressure exercises can also be practiced while you are at work, sitting in a chair. Sit back with your spine supported, feet flat on the floor, your eyes focused at a low point in front of you, and take several long deep breaths as you unobtrusively hold the points.

Deep Relaxation Guide

Close your eyes and feel your body relax. Wiggle your toes, letting them relax. Rotate your feet so your ankles relax. Gently move your legs, feeling your calves, knees, and thighs relax. . . . Now tighten your buttocks muscles; let them relax. . . . Feel your abdominal organs and pelvic area relax. . . . Take several long, slow, deep breaths into your abdominal area, letting your belly relax. Whatever you are hanging on to inside your mind, just let it go . . . .

Let your whole back relax. . . . Relax your arms. . . . Feel each finger relax. . . . Tell your shoulders and neck to relax. . . . Let go of any tension in your forehead and eyebrows. . . . Let your temples and ears relax. . . . Lips, teeth, and tongue relax. . . . Gently move your jaw from side to side, letting it relax. . . . Relax your nose and your throat and tell your eyes to relax completely. . . . Finally, feel your whole body totally relax. Allow your thoughts to flow, letting your mind and body completely relax.

Your whole consciousness changes during deep relaxation. When you no longer have physical, muscular, or mental resistances, your mind is able to experience its oneness with the body — and perceive the interconnectedness of everything in life.

Now that you have an understanding of what acupressure is, how to find a point, and some of the ways that acupressure can be used, you are ready to help yourself take care of forty common ailments.

If you feel light-headed after an acupressure session, use caution and do not drive until you feel stable and fully alert.

3
Acne, Eczema, and Other Skin Problems

Skin disorders[8] that are caused or worsened by stress, nervous tension, or fatigue can be relieved by using acupressure's potent points. Acupressure enhances how we feel and how we look by releasing muscular tension and increasing circulation. There are many points that relieve acne, tone facial muscles, and improve the condition of the skin. Dr. Katsusuke Serizawa's medical research at Tokyo University proved that acupressure therapy can return body functions to normality, thereby relieving skin and muscular problems.[9]

Many skin disorders can be relieved by using the following acupressure formula combining three types of potent points: local, trigger, and tonic points. First, you use the local points to help increase circulation in the area where the skin has erupted. Next use trigger points to stimulate the organs and glands that govern skin functions. According to traditional Chinese medicine, those organs are primarily the lungs, large intestine, liver, and stomach.

Last, tonic points are used for overall rejuvenation. The tonic point located in the lower back strengthens the immune system, the kidneys, and the adrenal glands, which in turn fortifies the body's entire system. The tonic point not only helps people cope with the stress in their lives but also reinforces emotional stability, an important factor in relieving many skin disorders.

Acne

Acupressure's relaxing and soothing effects help clear up blemishes and pimples by easing the emotional distress and hormonal imbalances that often aggravate acne. After using acupressure to balance various functions of the body, Dr. Serizawa found that patients' pimples occurred less often.[10] Potent points such as Facial Beauty and Heavenly Appearance (illustrated later in this chapter) are especially helpful.

Complementary Therapy: Along with using acupressure, it is important to practice breathing exercises as well as aerobic exercise daily. Thoroughly cleaning the skin with antibacterial soap also helps prevent the infections.

Diet: From the perspective of Oriental dietary therapy, it is important to avoid sugar, dairy products (including ice cream), chocolate, coffee, and all rich, greasy foods.

Eczema

Eczema is a dry, itchy condition. The skin often becomes red and inflamed. Eczema produces dry scales that break open, releasing a watery fluid.

In Japan, there is an ancient belief that the skin reflects the condition of one's internal organs. When the internal organs are fatigued, the effect appears on the skin immediately.[11]

---

[8] Consult your physician about any marks that are changing color or behaving suspiciously.
[9] Katsusuke Serizawa, M.D., *Tsubo: Vital Points for Oriental Therapy* (Tokyo: Japan Publications, 1976), 38.

[10] Katsusuke Serizawa, M.D., *Tsubo: Vital Points,* 240.
[11] Katsusuke Serizawa, M.D., *Effective Tsubo Therapy* (Tokyo: Japan Publications, 1980), 37.

Complementary Therapy: In addition to using the following acupressure point routine two or three times daily, you can help resolve eczema by fortifying your system with traditional Oriental breathing exercises. For instance, stand with your arms by your sides. Inhale as your arms come up and over your head. Exhale as you lower your arms again. Repeat ten to twenty times.

Diet: Eliminate all shellfish, especially shrimp, crab, and lobster, from your diet. Eating plenty of dandelion greens in salads and making a tea out of the dandelion root, for instance, is also good for relieving eczema. Following are descriptions of how to use the tonic, trigger, and local points for relieving skin disorders.

Potent Points for Relieving Acne and Other Skin Disorders

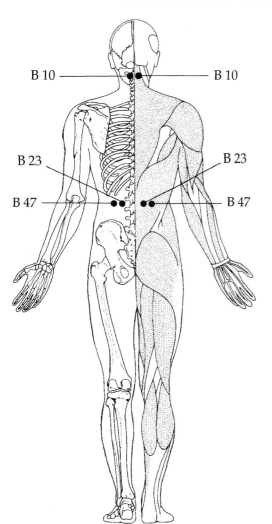

B 10 — B 10

B 23 — B 23

B 47 — B 47

Sea of Vitality (B 23 & B 47)

Caution: Do not press on disintegrating discs or fractured or broken bones. If you have a weak back, a few minutes of stationary, light touching instead of pressure can be very healing. See your doctor first if you have any questions or need medical advice.

Location: In the lower back (between the second and third lumbar vertebrae) two to four finger widths away from the spine at waist level.

Benefits: Relieves acne, eczema, and bruises on the body.

Three Mile Point (St 36)

Location: Four finger widths below the kneecap toward the outside of the shinbone.

Benefits: Strengthens and tones the muscles and improves the condition of the skin throughout the entire body.

Heavenly Pillar (B 10)

Location: One-half inch below the base of the skull on the ropy muscles one-half inch outward from either side of the spine.

Benefits: Relieves stress related to skin disorders such as acne.

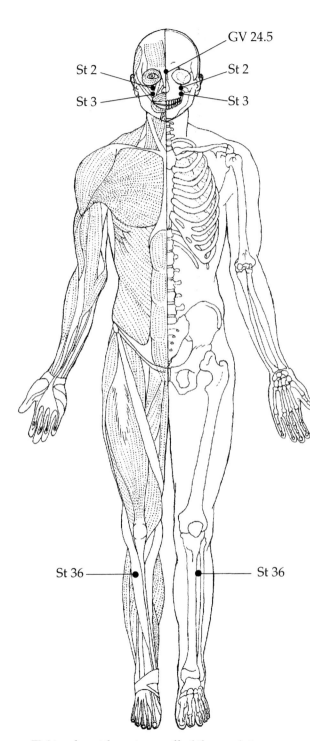

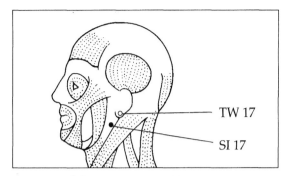

■ *You do not have to use all of these points. Using just one or two of them can be effective.*

Four Whites (St 2)

Location: One finger width below the lower ridge of the eye socket in line with the center of the iris in an indentation of the cheek.

Benefits: Remedies acne and facial blemishes.

Facial Beauty (St 3)

Location: At the bottom of the cheekbone, directly below the pupil.

Benefits: Relieves acne, facial blemishes, poor complexion, and sagging cheeks; and improves facial circulation.

Wind Screen (TW 17)

Location: In the indentation directly behind the ear lobe.

Benefits: Balances the thyroid gland to increase the luster of the skin; relieves hives.

Heavenly Appearance (SI 17)

Location: In the indentation directly below the ear lobe and behind the jawbone.

Benefits: Balances the thyroid gland to increase the luster of the skin; relieves hives.

Third Eye Point (GV 24.5)

Location: Directly between your eyebrows in the indentation where the bridge of the nose meets the center of the forehead.

Benefits: Stimulates the pituitary gland, which is the master endocrine gland, to enhance the condition of the skin throughout the body.

Potent Point Exercises

Sit up straight on the front edge of your chair.

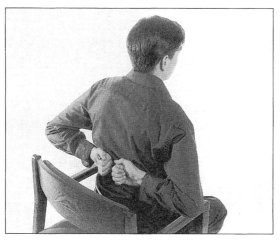

Step 1

Briskly rub B 23 and B 47: Use the backs of your hands to rub the lower back for one minute as you breathe deeply. This friction will stimulate both the inner and outer Sea of Vitality points at the same time.

Step 2

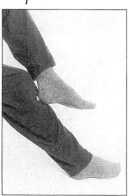

Briskly rub St 36: Use your heel to firmly rub the St 36 point on the opposite leg, below the outside of the knee. Place your heel one finger width outside of your shinbone. If you are on the correct spot, a muscle should flex as you move your foot up and down. Briskly rub this point for one minute. Then switch sides and stimulate St 36 on the opposite leg. This important tonic point fortifies the condition of the skin and is traditionally indicated for relieving eczema.

Sit comfortably against the back of your chair.

Step 3

Firmly press B 10: Grasp the back of your neck with one hand, using all of your fingers on one side and the heel of your hand on the other side to firmly squeeze the ropy neck muscles. This potent point benefits the skin as well as the nervous system.

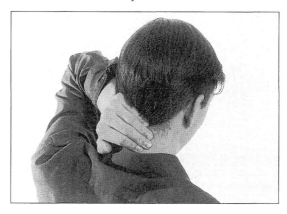

Step 4

Firmly but gently press St 2 and St 3 on your cheeks for relieving facial blemishes. Hold these points for one minute, pressing firmly enough to feel just a slight pressure in your eyes.

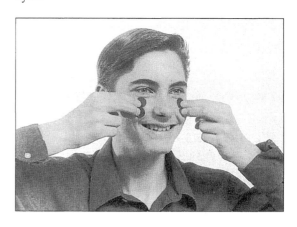

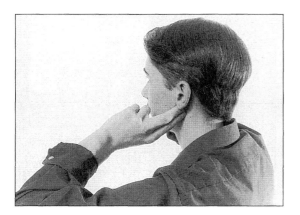

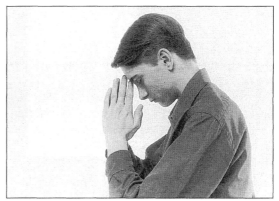

Step 5

Lightly press TW 17 and SI 17 using your middle and index fingertips to press directly underneath your earlobes and breathe deeply for one minute. These points are usually very tender.

Step 6

Touch GV 24.5: Bring your palms together and use your middle and index fingers to lightly touch the Third Eye point. Concentrate your attention on the point and breathe deeply for two minutes.

Additional Points for Acne, Eczema, and Other Skin Problems

For illustrations of related points for relieving acne and other skin problems, see chapter 4, "Allergies"; chapter 14, "Depression and Emotional Balancing"; and chapter 40, "Swelling and Water Retention."

4

ALLERGIES

$\mathcal{A}$n allergy is a sensitivity to a substance; material; or particular food, plant, or animal. Some of the more common allergic reactions include dizziness, headaches, hay fever, fatigue, difficulty breathing, constipation, stomach cramps, fever, hives, and depression. There are many types of allergy, some of which are inherited. Acupressure, while not a cure, can be an effective method for relieving many symptoms of allergic reactions by balancing the body's systems once you and your doctor have established the cause and seriousness of your allergy.[12]

Because allergy symptoms are so varied, there is no practical way in one chapter to cover how to use acupressure for each specific minor allergic reaction such as wheezing, itching, and bloodshot eyes. Instead, this chapter presents a general point sequence that can help balance and stabilize your body when you have a reaction and also strengthen you to prevent future reactions.

Janet, a client of mine and a recently retired social worker, suffered constantly from allergies, always wheezing, coughing, and blowing her nose. Janet was extremely fatigued from a recent trip to England, where she had contracted a sinus infection. Strange, warm winds the previous two nights had also stirred up her allergies, causing redness in her eyes and nasal congestion. Although she had gotten a prescription for penicillin, she preferred not to take it. I showed Janet how to press several points for decongestion (see page 26). I recommended that she practice these points at least three times a day. She used a relaxation audiotape to re-balance her system further from the stress of traveling. Two weeks later Janet called me to report that her coughing, sneezing, and nasal congestion had subsided almost completely. "I don't think I've felt this healthy and relaxed in years," she proclaimed. She has kept up her daily practice and now contracts far fewer colds.

The following points help relieve the symptoms and aftereffects of many allergic reactions. I've devised a "quick formula" — for a powerful combination of points to relieve allergy symptoms temporarily if your time is limited. Otherwise, you should use these points in the longer routine. This routine can also be incorporated with other points found in other chapters associated with your specific problem. Although these points can be used occasionally to relieve the symptoms associated with allergies, it is best to practice the full point sequence routine on a daily basis.

---

[12] **Caution:** Serious allergic reactions that may lead to complications should be seen immediately by a physician. This chapter should not be used as a substitute for medication or treatment of an allergy for which you are under a doctor's care or may need to be.

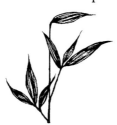

Potent Points for Relieving Allergies

Joining the Valley (Hoku) (LI 4)

Caution: This point is forbidden for pregnant women unless they are in labor because its stimulation can cause premature contractions in the uterus.

Location: In the webbing between your thumb and index finger. On the outside of the hand, find the highest spot of the muscle when the thumb and index fingers are brought close together.

Benefits: Relieves all kinds of allergies, such as headaches, hay fever, sneezing, and itching.

Bigger Rushing (Lv 3)

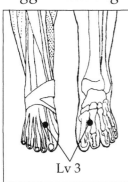

Lv 3

Location: On the top of the foot in the valley between the big toe and the second toe.

Benefits: Relieves all kinds of allergic reactions, especially bloodshot eyes and neuromuscular disorders.

Quick Formula for Relieving Allergies

Step 1:

This step should be skipped if you are pregnant.
Firmly press LI 4: Open your left hand in front of you, with the palm facing down. LI 4, an antihistamine point, is located in the center of the webbing between your thumb and index finger. Place your right thumb on top in the middle of the webbing with your right index finger underneath the palm and apply pressure by squeezing into the webbing. Angle the pressure toward the bone that

connects with the index finger. Take several long, slow, deep breaths as you firmly press into this point. Then press LI 4 on your right hand with your left thumb and index finger. Breath deeply and hold the point for one minute.

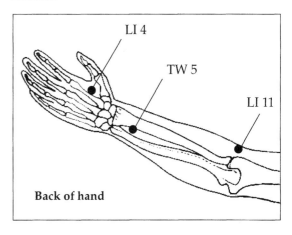

Back of hand

Step 2:

Stimulate point Lv 3: Use your index fingers to press in between the bones on the top of your feet between the large toe and the second toe. Firmly rub in the troughs and angle the pressure toward the bone that connects with the second toe to stimulate this important point for counteracting allergies.

Outer Gate (TW 5)

Location: On the top of the forearm between the two armbones, two and one-half finger widths above the wrist crease.

Benefits: Relieves allergic reactions by strengthening the immune system.

Crooked Pond (LI 11)

Location: On the top, outer end of the elbow crease.

Benefits: Relieves allergies, particularly inflamed skin disorders (such as hives and rashes), itching, and fevers.

Heavenly Pillar (B 10)

Location: One-half inch below the base of the skull, on the ropy muscles one-half inch outward from either side of the spine.

Benefits: Relieves allergic reactions such as exhaustion, headache, and swollen eyes.

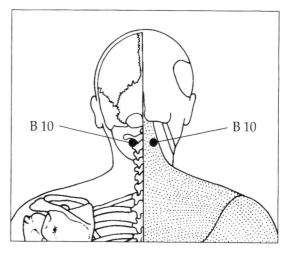

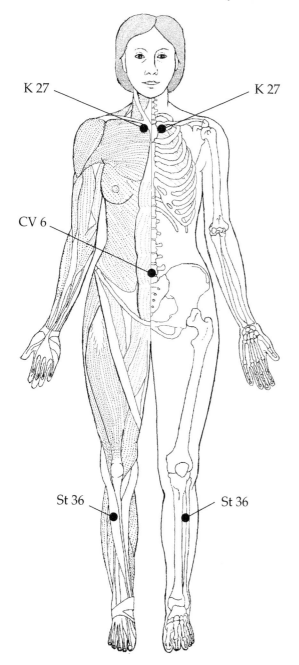

Elegant Mansion (K 27)

Location: In the hollow below the collarbone next to the breastbone.

Benefits: Relieves allergies associated with chest congestion, breathing difficulties, asthma, coughing, and sore throats.

Sea of Energy (CV 6)

Location: Two finger widths directly below the belly button.

Benefits: Relieves allergies that accompany constipation, gas, fatigue, general weakness, and insomnia.

Three Mile Point (St 36)

Location: Four finger widths below the kneecap on the outside of the leg.

Benefits: Strengthens the whole body to prevent as well as relieve allergies.

■ *You do not have to use all of these points. Using just one or two of them whenever you have a free hand can be effective.*

Potent Point Exercises

Sit comfortably in a chair for the following acupressure routine.

Step 1

Stimulate point TW 5: Use your thumb to rub and press TW 5, two and one-half finger widths above the outer wrist crease.

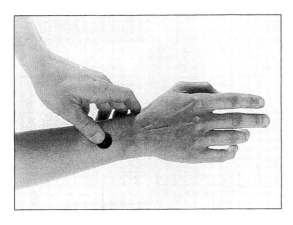

Step 2

Firmly press LI 11: Bend your arm and place your opposite thumb at the end of the elbow crease at the joint. Firmly press for a few seconds and then release; repeat five to ten times. Then switch sides and repeat the firm pressure five more times.

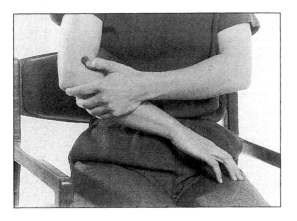

Step 3

Firmly hold B 10: Use your fingertips and the heel of your hand to firmly grasp hold of the muscles on both sides of the back of your neck for one minute.

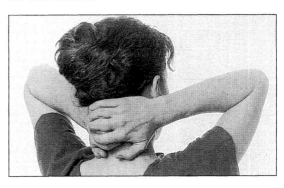

Step 4

Press K 27: First, place your fingertips on the two knobs of your collarbone below your throat. Then move directly down to the first indentation. Press firmly into these hollow areas for one full minute, taking long, slow, deep breaths.

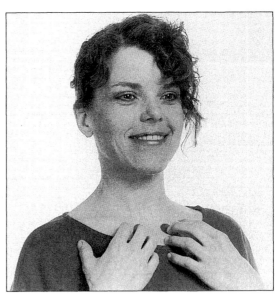

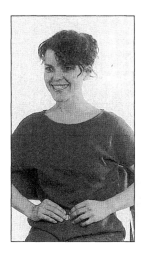

Step 5
Firmly hold CV 6:
Place your fingertips two inches directly below your belly button. Press one to two inches deep inside your abdomen for one minute as you take long, deep breaths.

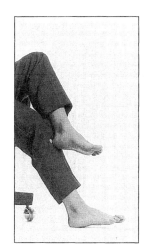

Step 6
Briskly rub St 36:
Place your right heel on St 36 of your left leg. If you are on the correct spot, a muscle should pop out as you flex your foot up and down. Briskly rub it for one minute. Do the same on the other side to help prevent further allergies.

Additional Points for Relieving Allergies

For illustrations of related points for relieving allergies, see chapter 10, "Chronic Fatigue Syndrome"; chapter 23, "Immune System Boosting"; and chapter 38, "Sinus Problems and Hay Fever."

5

ANKLE AND FOOT PROBLEMS

*B*ecause we depend on our ankles to support our weight, it is difficult to stand and move when they feel painful and stiff. The whole body is thrown out of balance. Weak ankles place undue stress on the hips and knees, which can eventually lead to degenerative osteoarthritis. Local acupressure points in the ankles are effective for relieving ankle pain, swelling, and stiffness. You should always apply pressure to these points gradually. You can also use them to strengthen the ankle joint, which can help prevent such problems. If you have strained or sprained an ankle, however, let it rest as much as possible for two or three weeks to enable healing in addition to using the potent points in this chapter.

I sprained my ankle several years ago, and it would not heal completely. It was stiff and ached a lot, especially in the morning. Because the joint was weak and vulnerable, I resprained it several times that year. Finally, after several months went by, I disciplined myself to hold point GB 40 on the ankle for fifteen minutes, twice a day. After just one week, the pain and stiffness disappeared. And, because I continue to press it daily, the joint is stronger and I haven't sprained my ankle in years.

People who have weak, swollen, inflexible ankles often avoid sports and other vigorous physical activities such as hiking or even walking. An inactive person is more prone to excessive weight gain, and this creates additional stress on the joint. This in turn makes it harder for an inactive person to become more active. Self-acupressure techniques enable you to strengthen the joint and reduce swelling, so that you can pursue a wide range of physical activities in your daily life.

One of my clients, a physical therapist in her forties named Sylvia, had injured her knee and could not participate in her regular physical exercise program. She was feeling depressed about the weight she had gained and the problems that had occurred with her husband. Sylvia's feet and ankles were puffy from standing too much on the job. I worked on her legs and feet, particularly emphasizing the acupressure points illustrated on page 32. At the end of the session, the ankle and foot swelling were gone, and she felt tremendously relaxed.

The following acupressure points can help you relieve ankle swelling, pain, and pressure; promote healing after a sprain; and strengthen a weak ankle.

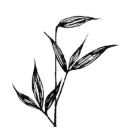

Potent Points for Relieving Ankle Problems

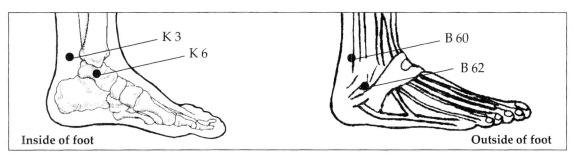

Inside of foot · Outside of foot

Bigger Stream (K 3)

Caution: This point is forbidden to be strongly stimulated after the third month of pregnancy.

Location: In the hollow midway between the protrusion of the inside anklebone and the Achilles tendon, which joins the back of the calf to the back of the heel.

Benefits: Relieves swollen feet and ankle pain, and strengthens the ankle joint.

High Mountains (B 60)

Location: Opposite K 3, in the hollow between the outer anklebone and the Achilles tendon.

Benefits: Relieves swollen feet, ankle pains, thigh pain, rheumatism in the foot joints, and lower back pain.

Illuminated Sea (K 6)

Location: One thumb width below the inside of the anklebone.

Benefits: Relieves swollen ankles, as well as heel and ankle pain.

Calm Sleep (B 62)

Location: In the first indentation directly below the outer anklebone. This hollow is one-third the distance from the outer anklebone to the bottom of the heel.

Benefits: Relieves heel pain, ankle pain, insomnia, and general foot pains.

Ankle Sprains

Ankle sprains are common among athletes. The following point on the outside of the foot, called Wilderness Mound, is very effective for relieving ankle sprains. Hold this point for five to ten minutes, alternating every sixty seconds between light and firm pressure. Complete the routine with a minute of light touch, without pressure. For maximum healing benefit, hold until you feel an even pulse in the area.

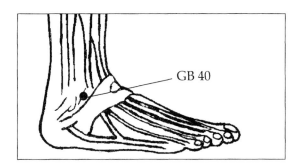

Wilderness Mound (GB 40)

Location: In the large hollow directly in front of the outer anklebone.

Benefits: Relieves ankle sprain, toe cramps, and sciatic pain that travels into the side of the foot.

■ *You do not have to use all of these points. Using just one or two of them whenever you have a free hand can be effective.*

Potent Point Exercises

Lie down on your back or sit comfortably.

Step 1

Firmly press K 3 with B 60: Bend your right leg, placing your right foot on your left knee. Use your left thumb on your right ankle, gradually applying pressure to K 3 (on the inside of the ankle). Use your fingertips to press B 60 (on the outside of the ankle) in an indentation between the anklebone and the Achilles tendon. Firmly hold for one to two minutes, angling your finger pressure underneath your ankle bone. Then switch and use your right hand on your left ankle.

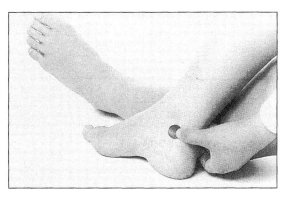

Step 2

Stimulate K 6 and B 62: Gently grasp both K 6 (inside ankle) and B 62 (outside ankle) directly below the anklebone. Hold firmly for ten seconds and then slowly release. Repeat five to ten times on each ankle.

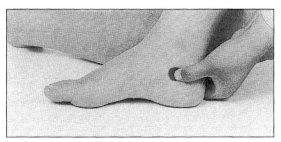

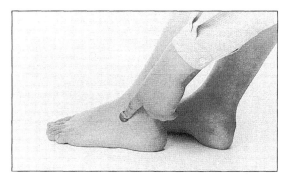

Step 3

Hold GB 40: Press slowly but firmly into GB 40 (the large indentation in the front of the outer anklebone). Hold this important ankle strengthening point three to five minutes or until you feel a well-defined pulse. Then hold this point on your other side until you feel a pulse.

Step 4

Relaxation: After stimulating these ankle points, take a few minutes to close your eyes and relax or give yourself the following wonderful foot massage.

Foot Massage

This foot massage stimulates a series of acupressure and reflexology points in the feet and ankles to restore and stimulate your body's natural energy system.

Begin by slipping off your shoes. Place your left ankle on your right knee, so you can comfortably reach your left foot. Place both thumbs on the bottom of your foot near your toes, with your fingers on the top of your foot. Thoroughly massage your toes, as you take a nice deep breath. Next, firmly walk your thumbs back along the sole of your foot, pressing all parts of the bottom of your foot as you massage gradually toward your heel. Focus on taking long, slow, deep breaths as you thoroughly massage the sole of your foot. Now use your thumbs to massage the arch of the foot, starting at the heel, slowly working your hands up to the base of your large toe.

Use your fingertips to press gently between the bones on the top of your foot, as you press the bottom of your foot with your thumbs. Next, move your hands to your ankle, thoroughly massaging both sides of your Achilles tendon all the way up to the base of your calf muscle. Now switch legs and massage your other foot.

Additional Points for Ankle and Foot Problems

For illustrations of related points for relieving ankle problems, see chapter 7, "Arthritis and Nonarticular Rheumatism"; chapter 28, "Knee Pain"; and chapter 40, "Swelling and Water Retention."

6
ANXIETY AND NERVOUSNESS

*M*any acupressure points relieve anxiety and nervousness by relaxing you and increasing circulation throughout the body. When tension is released and you feel better physically, you also feel better about yourself and can gain a new perspective on the conflicts or issues that underlie your anxiety.

Dorothy, an administrative assistant, suffered from panic attacks and nervousness. She was anxious about how much weight she had gained, her job and the family's financial difficulties, and her son who suffered from asthma attacks. Immediately after receiving her fourth acupressure session she felt relaxed and centered. After two months of treatment she had made great strides in managing her weight[13] and her morale had visibly improved.

As you do the following acupressure routines and deep breathing exercises, be aware of thoughts and feelings that surface. Because the practices are deeply relaxing, they often trigger a chain of new insights that can help overcome anxiety or nervousness.

Anxiety Attacks

Anxiety (which comes from the Latin root meaning "twisted rope"[14]) is an all-too-common result of the stress of modern life. When an anxiety attack occurs you can hold the Sea of Tranquility point (CV 17) on the center of your breastbone for relief. Concentrate on breathing slowly and deeply while holding it to increase its calming effect. The other points illustrated in this chapter can be used to strengthen and balance your system and to prevent nervous attacks. It is advisable to see a holistic medical doctor or a therapist if your anxiety is not relieved after practicing the following points and deep breathing exercises twenty minutes, twice a day for a week.

The Importance of Deep Breathing

You can learn to relieve your anxiety in just a few minutes by focusing on how you breathe. Long, deep breathing is important for releasing tension as well as for emotional balancing. The next time you are nervous or anxious, check out how you are breathing. When you are anxious your breathing will often be shallow. If you increase the depth and capacity of your breath, you can relieve your nervousness.

Sometimes it's difficult to breathe deeply due to a number of emotional factors: constriction in the chest due to emotional pain or anxiety, great grief or sadness, holding on to an unfulfilled expectation, or even a physical disability. Try the deep relaxation exercise described in this chapter and make time to practice the breathing techniques regularly. You will begin to feel better.

Lifestyle

Get plenty of daily exercise, including stretching, breathing, and aerobic exercises such as swimming, biking, dancing, or running.

Diet

Avoid refined foods made with white flour and sugar as well as coffee and foods that have a high salt content.

---

[13] Michael Reed Gach, *For Women Only: Weight Loss* (New York: Simon & Schuster Audio Division, 1989).
[14] Gerald Epstein, M.D., *Healing Visualizations* (New York: Bantam Books, 1989), p. 59.

Potent Points for Relieving Anxiety and Nervousness

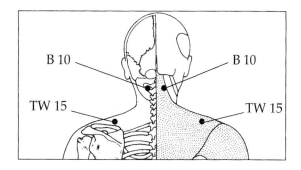

Heavenly Rejuvenation (TW 15)

Location: On the shoulders, midway between the base of the neck and the outside of the shoulders, one-half inch below the top of the shoulders.

Benefits: Relieves nervous tension and stiff necks; increases resistance to colds and flus; and is good for the lungs.

Heavenly Pillar (B 10)

Location: One finger width below the base of the skull on the ropy muscles one-half inch outward from the spine.

Benefits: Relieves stress, overexhaustion, insomnia, heaviness in the head, eyestrain, stiff necks, swollen eyes, and sore throats.

Crooked Marsh (P 3)

Location: On the inside of the arm at the lower end of the elbow crease when the arm is bent.

Benefits: Relieves nervous stomaches, anxiety, arm pain, elbow pain, and chest discomfort.

Inner Gate (P 6)

Location: In the middle of the inner side of the forearm two and one-half finger widths from the wrist crease.

Benefits: Relieves nausea, anxiety, palpitations, and wrist pain.

Spirit Gate (H 7)

Location: On the little finger side of the forearm at the crease of the wrist.

Benefits: Relieves emotional imbalances, fear, nervousness, anxiety, and forgetfulness.

Third Eye Point (GV 24.5)

Location: Directly between the eyebrows, in the indentation where the bridge of the nose meets the forehead.

Benefits: Calms the body to relieve nervousness.

Sea of Tranquility (CV 17)

Location: On the center of the breastbone, three thumb widths up from the base of the bone.

Benefits: Relieves nervousness, anxiety, chest tension, anguish, depression, hysteria, and other emotional imbalances.

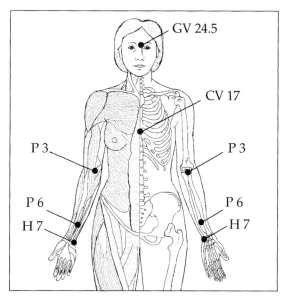

■ *You do not have to use all of these points. Using just one or two of them whenever you have a free hand can be effective.*

Potent Point Exercises

Step 1

Upholding Heaven: A Breathing Exercise

Stand with your feet comfortably apart and your arms at your sides. Inhale, raising your arms, palms up, out to the sides and then up above your head.

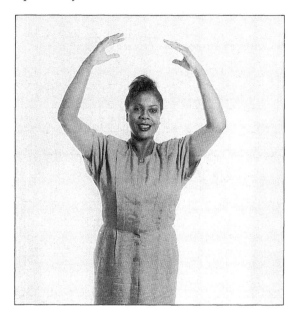

Interlock your fingers, with your palms facing each other. Turn your palms inside out so that your palms face the sky. Inhale, and gently stretch farther upward, with your head tilted back.

Exhale, lowering your chin to your chest and letting your arms float back down to your sides. Repeat five times.

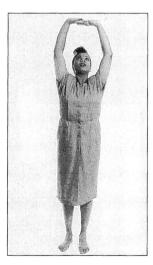

Continue steps 2 through 5 sitting comfortably.

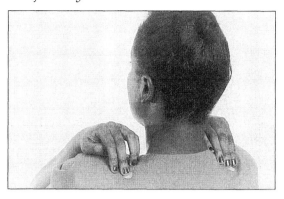

Step 2

Press both TW 15 points: Curving your fingers, hook your right hand on your right shoulder, your left hand on your left shoulder. Close your eyes. With your fingertips, firmly press TW 15 on the top of your shoulders and take three long, slow, deep breaths. Then relax your hands into your lap, taking another few long, slow, deep breaths.

Step 3

Firmly press B 10: Again, curve your fingers, hooking your fingertips on the ropy muscles of the neck. Press firmly while you take three more long, slow, deep breaths. Then relax your hands back into your lap.

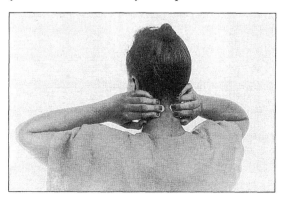

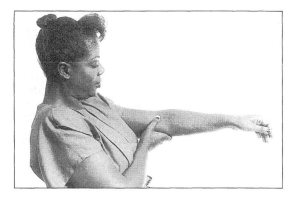

Step 4

Hold P 3; press P 6 and H 7: Hold P 3 with your thumb (see photo above). Press P 6 and H 7 with your index and middle fingers for thirty to sixty seconds each (see point locations on page 36). Then switch sides. If you continue to breathe deeply through your nose, you will find that your body is releasing its stress and nervous tension.

Step 5

Touch GV 24.5: Close your eyes and bring your palms together. Use your middle and index fingers to lightly touch the Third Eye Point between your eyebrows. Close your eyes and take long, slow, deep breaths as you concentrate on this point for a full minute.

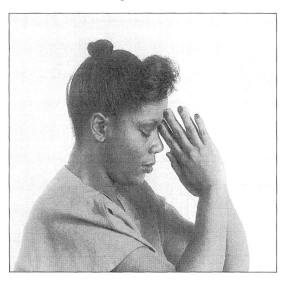

Step 6

Press CV 17: Keeping your palms together, use the back of your thumbs against your breastbone to press CV 17 firmly, at the level of your heart. Continue to keep your eyes closed and concentrate on breathing slow, even, deep breaths into your heart to completely dispel any anxiety.

Focus on breathing deeply for two more minutes. Gently control your respiratory system, making each breath grow longer and deeper than the last one. Breathe out any tensions you feel restricting your lungs from moving fully and naturally. Feel your mind clear with each breath.

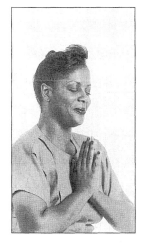

Notice the resistance your mind creates: the worries and judgments it comes up against. Take several deep breaths and dissolve these barriers. Breathe deeply and gently, remembering that you are breathing in life itself.

Hold the breath at the top of the exhalation for a moment, feeling its fullness. Then exhale smoothly, letting your hands drift down into your lap, and relax, feeling the vitality of the breath circulate throughout your body.

Additional Points for Relieving Anxiety and Nervousness

For illustrations of related points for relieving anxiety, see chapter 8, "Asthma and Breathing Difficulties"; chapter 14, "Depression and Emotional Balancing"; chapter 26, "Irritability, Frustration, and Dealing With Change."

7

ARTHRITIS AND NONARTICULAR RHEUMATISM

*O*ne of my favorite students, Leslie, a fifty-eight-year-old widow, was searching for a drug-free way to relieve the pain and swelling of the arthritis in her hands and toes, as well as a variety of allergies. She had lost feeling in her toes, and her doctor had said that she had very slight chance of regaining feeling in them. After three months of acupressure treatments every week, she was able to flex her toes back and forth, and move them at will without pain. Slowly, feeling came back into her toes. I will never forget how excited Leslie was to be able to wiggle her toes.

The special potent points in this chapter, when held properly for several minutes every day, can relieve muscle aches and arthritic pain, increase the mobility of your joints, strengthen them, and prevent further joint deterioration.

There are over 100 different types of arthritis. With some types, such as chronic rheumatoid arthritis, it will take longer to increase joint mobility and become pain free. Most people with arthritis will need to practice these self-acupressure techniques two to three times a day for six months and continue once a day for prevention and health maintenance.

Acupressure is especially effective for relieving nonarticular (nonjoint-related) rheumatism. This soft-tissue condition, also referred to as *myofibrosis* or *fibrositis*, has symptoms similar to rheumatoid arthritis, such as morning stiffness, muscle tenderness, debilitating fatigue, and often depression.

As Dr. Murray C. Sokoloff has stated, "Easily reversible conditions such as fibromyalgia, fibrositis, and myofascial syndrome may go into complete remission with the help of acupressure treatments. Acupressure offers relief with no risk and at the same time is inexpensive and easily integrated into one's life."[15]

Medical doctors have found that patients who suffer from fibrositis, a disorder involving musculoskeletal pain and aching, especially in the morning, numbness, disturbed sleep, and fatigue, have tender areas that researchers have termed "tender points."[16] These tender spots on the body correspond to acupressure points used in traditional Chinese medicine. If you have arthritis, you can easily locate many of these points simply by pressing the areas where the pain concentrates. When you find the area, instead of massaging, rubbing, or kneading, simply hold it firmly for a few minutes. If it is extremely sensitive, gradually decrease the pressure until you find a balance between pain and pleasure.

Norman Shealy, M.D., a world-renowned pain specialist and director of the pain rehabilitation center in La Crosse, Wisconsin, has found several acupressure points to be useful in treating pain and has incorporated them into his overall pain reduction program, which can be used for arthritis pain.[17]

---

[15] Murray C. Sokoloff, M.D., "Foreword." In *Arthritis Relief at Your Fingertips*, by Michael Reed Gach (New York: Warner Books, 1989), viii.

[16] Hugh Smythe, M.D., "Fibrositis," *American Journal of Medicine*, 81, no. 3A (1986): 2-6.

[17] Norman Shealy, M.D., *The Pain Game* (Berkeley: Celestial Arts, 1976), 95.

Acupressure is also extremely effective in reducing the inflammation that accompanies arthritis. The potent points presented in this chapter are selected from twelve anti-inflam- matory points.[18] If stimulated on a regular, daily basis, they increase circulation, which in turn reduces inflammation and at the same time increases joint mobility.

Potent Points for Relieving Arthritis

Joining the Valley (Hoku) (LI 4)
Caution: This point is forbidden for pregnant women until labor because its stimulation can cause premature contractions in the uterus.

Location: In the webbing between the thumb and index finger at the highest spot of the muscle when the thumb and index finger are brought close together.

Benefits: Relieves pain and inflammation in the hand, wrist, elbow, shoulder, and neck.

Outer Gate (TW 5)
Location: Two and one-half finger widths above the wrist crease on the outer forearm midway between the two bones of the arm.

Benefits: Relieves rheumatism, tendonitis, wrist pain, and shoulder pain.

Three Mile Point (St 36)

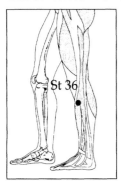

Location: Four finger widths below the kneecap, one finger width to the outside of the leg.

Benefits: Strengthens the body, benefits the joints, and relieves the fatigue that often results from the drain of dealing with arthritic pain.

Crooked Pond (LI 11)
Location: On the upper edge of the elbow crease.

Benefits: Relieves arthritic pain, especially in the elbow and shoulder.

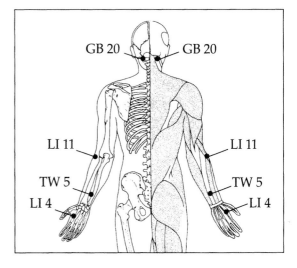

Gates of Consciousness (GB 20)
Location: Below the base of the skull, in the hollow between the two large, vertical neck muscles, two to three inches apart depending on the size of the head.

Benefits: Relieves arthritis, as well as the following common complaints that often accompany arthritic pain: headaches, insomnia, stiff neck, neck pain, fatigue, and general irritability.

■ *You do not have to use all of these points. Using just one or two of them whenever you have a free hand can be effective.*

---

[18] For more information on how to use these acupressure points to relieve arthritic pain see Michael Reed Gach, *Arthritis Relief at Your Fingertips* (London: Piatkus Books, 1989), 27-38.

Potent Point Exercises

Sit comfortably for the following routine.

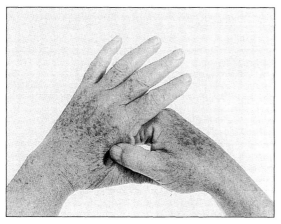

Step 1

Press into LI 4: To press this anti-inflammatory point on your left hand, place your right thumb into the webbing between the thumb and index finger to gradually direct pressure underneath the bone that attaches to your index finger. Press for a couple of minutes while breathing deeply, then switch hands and work on your right hand.

Step 2

Press TW 5: To find this point, place the knuckles of your left hand on top of your right forearm two-and-one-half finger widths from the wrist crease. Use your knuckles to apply firm pressure on this point as you breathe deeply for one minute. Switch hands and work on your left arm.

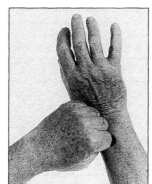

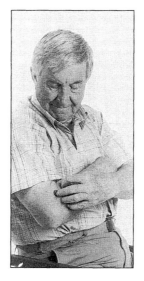

Step 3

Press LI 11: Bend your right arm in front of you with your palm facing down. To find this point, place the fingertips of your left hand on top of the right arm where the elbow crease ends. Press into the elbow joint firmly with your left fingers as your breathe deeply for one minute. Then switch sides and work on your left elbow.

Step 4

Firmly press GB 20: Place both of your thumbs underneath the base of your skull, two to three inches apart, into two hollow areas. Apply pressure gradually, as you slowly tilt your head back. Firmly press up and underneath the skull for one minute.

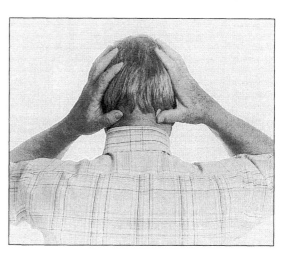

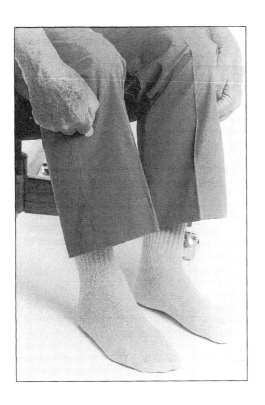

Step 5

Firmly press St 36: This is one of the most effective acupressure points for counteracting pain and fatigue. To find the point, measure four finger widths below your kneecap, placing your fingertips one-half inch outside the shinbone. If you're on the correct spot, a muscle should flex as you move your foot up and down a few times. Now make two fists and place them slightly to the outside of both legs just below your knees. Use your fists to briskly massage up and down along the outside of your shinbones for one minute. This rejuvenates the whole system.

For best results, practice this arthritis relief routine twice a day. If time does not permit, two applications a week will still have a beneficial effect.

Additional Points for Relieving Arthritis

For illustrations of related points for relieving arthritis pain, see chapter 9, "Backache and Sciatica"; chapter 13, "Cramps and Spasms"; chapter 20, "Headaches and Migraines"; chapter 28, "Knee Pain"; chapter 33, "Neck Tension, Whiplash, and Pain"; chapter 35, "Pain"; chapter 37, "Shoulder Tension"; and chapter 42, "Wrist Pain."

8
Asthma and Breathing Difficulties

$\mathcal{B}$reathing difficulties can cause the body to become toxic, sluggish, and incapable of healing. All of the cells, organs, and systems of our body need oxygen to carry out their functions.

Acupressure points on the upper chest, directly below the protrusions of your collarbone, held for just a few minutes, are particularly effective in restoring regular breathing. Others have been found helpful in increasing lung capacity, relaxing the large muscle groups connected to the respiratory system for easy breathing, and rejuvenating the lungs.

Asthma

A person with asthma experiences difficulty breathing, tightness in the chest, wheezing, and may cough up mucus. The walls of the bronchial tubes spasm and the air passages narrow, making it hard to exhale. Emotional stress, hormonal imbalances, and minor infections can make a person more susceptible to allergic reactions and asthma attacks. But you can often open these passages simply by relaxing the muscles in the bronchi by working on the potent points illustrated in this chapter.

A preliminary (unpublished) research study conducted by the Acupressure Institute in Berkeley, California, found that four out of the five of the adult asthmatic patients tested had a 20 percent increase in their vital lung capacity immediately after receiving twenty minutes of acupressure. The potent points illustrated in this chapter were the primary points used in the Institute's study.

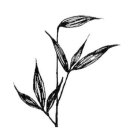

Potent Points for Relieving Asthma and Breathing Difficulties

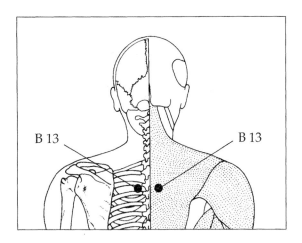

Elegant Mansion (K 27)

Location: In the hollow below the collarbone next to the breastbone.

Benefits: Relieves chest congestion, breathing difficulties, asthma, coughing, and anxiety.

Letting Go (Lu 1)

Location: On the outer part of the chest, three finger widths below the collarbone.

Benefits: Relieves asthma, breathing difficulties, chest tension and congestion, coughing, and tension due to emotional distress.

Lung Associated Point (B 13)

Location: One finger width below the upper tip of the shoulder blade, between the spine and the scapula.

Benefits: Relieves asthma, coughing, sneezing, and severe muscle spasms in the shoulders and neck.

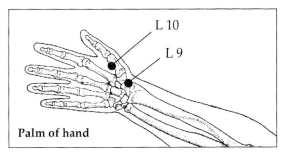

Palm of hand

Great Abyss (Lu 9)

Location: In the groove at the wrist fold below the base of the thumb.

Benefits: Relieves lung problems, coughing, and asthma.

Fish Border (Lu 10)

Location: On the palm side of the hand in the center of the pad at the base of the thumb.

Benefits: Relieves shallow breathing, coughing, and swollen throat.

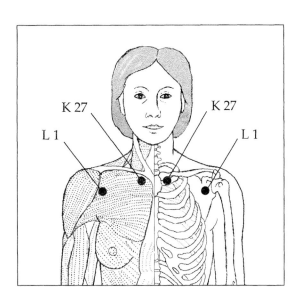

■ *You do not have to use all of these points. Using just one or two of them whenever you have a free hand can be effective.*

Potent Point Exercises

Sit up comfortably for the following acupressure routine.

Step 1

Firmly press B 13: Bring your right hand over your left shoulder to find point B 13 between the tip of your shoulder blade and your spine. Curve your fingers to hook into tension in this area. Take five long, deep breaths as you continue to firmly hold this point. Then switch sides, and take five additional deep breaths to hold B 13 on your other side.

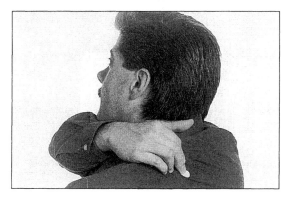

Step 2

Press both K 27 points: Use your thumbs to press the indentations directly below your collarbone. Apply gradual, firm pressure on both of these upper chest points as you take five more long, deep breaths.

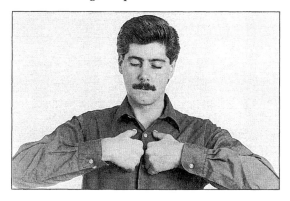

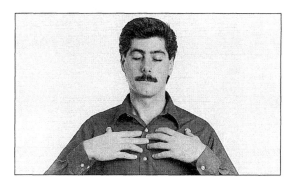

Step 3

Firmly press Lu 1: Make fists in front of your chest with your thumbs pointing up. Place your thumbs on the outer portion of your chest, pressing on the muscles that run horizontally below your collarbone. Find a knot or sensitive spot on the chest muscles. Underneath that knot is Lu 1, an important acupressure point for breathing difficulties. Let your head hang forward toward your chest, relaxing your neck, as you maintain firm pressure on those muscles with your thumbs. Continue to hold this point while breathing deeply for two minutes.

Step 4

Hold Lu 9 and Lu 10: First find Lu 9, in the indentation of the wrist crease beneath the base of the thumb. After a few long, slow, deep breaths, move to Lu 10 in the center of

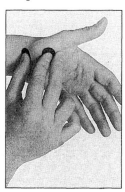

the base of your thumb. Continue to hold Lu 10 as you take several deep breaths. Then make a fist with your opposite hand to stimulate both of these points by lightly rubbing them briskly. After a minute or so, repeat the same points on the other hand.

A Deep Breathing Exercise

1. Lie flat on your back and reach up toward the sky with both hands. Take a deep breath, then as you hold your breath make tight fists and squeeze, tightening all the muscles in your arms.

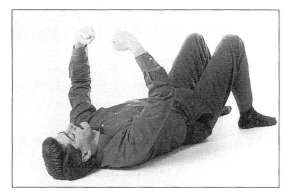

2. Slowly exhale, and keep tensing your arms as you bring your fists down toward your chest, with your elbows out to your sides.
3. Release your fists, and as you inhale once again stretch both your arms up toward the sky.
4. Make tight fists and again tense your arm muscles as you exhale, pulling your fists down toward your chest, as if you're pulling healing energy directly into your lungs.

After practicing this exercise several times, close your eyes, let your arms rest at your sides with your palms facing up, and just relax. As you breathe deeply, visualize healing energy circulating throughout your body.

Additional Points for Relieving Asthma

For illustrations of related points for relieving asthma and other breathing difficulties, see chapter 11, "Colds and Flu"; chapter 14, "Depression and Emotional Balancing"; and chapter 26, "Irritability, Frustration, and Dealing with Change."

9
BACKACHE AND SCIATICA

One of my clients, Ginger, is a retail store manager who suffered from severe lower-back pain. She complained about being tired and overweight. I held points on her legs and feet that worked on her lower back. After the acupressure session, as Ginger was slowly getting up, we heard her back crack. When the back muscles relax, the vertebrae often naturally fall into alignment. After just this one acupressure session, she felt much more relaxed, and the pain in her lower back was almost completely gone.

Back problems are one of the most common ailments in our society. Four out of five people have had severe back pain at least once in their lives.[19] The majority of sciatica and lower-back problems are related to stress, poor posture, accidents, or weak abdominal muscles. Back muscle or ligament strains are possible causes as well, so it is extremely important to keep your spine and back muscles strong and flexible. Acupressure is highly effective for relieving the muscular tension associated with lower-back pain and sciatica.

When your hip hurts or your lower back aches, your body automatically compensates for this weakness by taking pressure off that area and shifting it to another. This, unfortunately, shifts an extra burden to another area of your back, compounding the problem.

The effectiveness of acupressure can be enhanced by a healthy diet and the proper use of heat. According to traditional Chinese medicine, eating too much salt; drinking too much liquid; eating excessively cold foods as well as catching cold; and an excess of jarring exercise, fear, or paranoia can cause problems in the lower back area. My eighteen years of experience administering acupressure have confirmed this advice time and again. I would also suggest that you regularly practice gentle back care exercises to prevent back problems.

Using a heating pad, hot water bottle, or hot bath (if there is no inflammation) can also be helpful because heat provides *temporary* relief from stiffness and pain. But when you use heat in conjunction with acupressure on a muscular problem, the relief from tension and pain often lasts longer.

Caution: Do not press on disintegrating discs or on fractured or broken bones. For severe lower-back or sciatic pain, you must always first consult a medical or osteopathic doctor, chiropractor, or physical therapist.

---

[19] Michael Reed Gach, *The Bum Back Book* (Berkeley: Celestial Arts, 1985), 5.

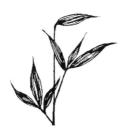

Potent Points for Relieving Lower-Back Aches

The following potent points stimulate the lower back to strengthen and heal it. The point behind the knee (B 54) is a special trigger point for alleviating lower-back pain. The Sea of Vitality points (B 23 and B 47) in the lower back and the Sea of Energy point (CV 6) in the lower abdomen help relieve back pain and especially benefit the kidneys and the urore-productive system. The Womb and Vitals point (B 48) in the buttocks is an effective lower-back and sciatic pain point. You can use any of these points separately or together in sequence for a more complete routine for relieving sciatica and lower-back aches.

Sea of Vitality (B 23 and B 47)

Caution: If you have a weak back, the Sea of Vitality points may be quite tender. In this case a few minutes of light, stationary touch instead of deep pressure can be very healing. See your doctor first if you have any questions or need medical advice.

Location: In the lower back (between the second and third lumbar vertebrae) two to four finger widths away from the spine at waist level.

Benefits: Relieves lower-back aches, sciatica, and the fatigue that often results from the pain.

Womb and Vitals (B 48)

Location: One to two finger widths outside the sacrum (the large bony area at the base of the spine) and midway between the top of the hipbone (iliac crest) and the base of the buttock.

Benefits: Relieves lower-back aches, sciatica, pelvic tension, hip pain, and tension.

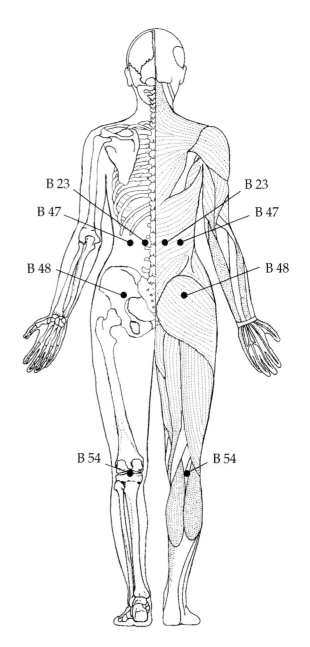

B 23 B 23
B 47 B 47
B 48 B 48
B 54 B 54

Sea of Energy (CV 6)

Location: Two finger widths directly below the belly button.

Benefits: Relieves lower-back weakness, tones weak abdominal muscles, and prevents a variety of lower-back problems.

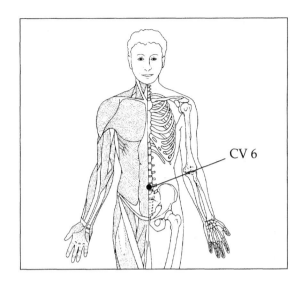

Commanding Middle (B 54)

Location: In the center of the back of the knee crease.

Benefits: Relieves back pain; sciatica; knee pain; back stiffness; and arthritis in the knees, back, and hips.

Potent Point Exercises

Begin this routine sitting and then lie down, as instructed, on a carpeted floor.

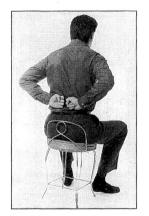

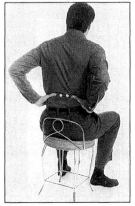

Step 1

Rub, then hold, B 23 and B 47: First, place the knuckles of both hands on your lower back, with your palms facing out. Rub your lower back with your knuckles vigorously enough to create warmth. Keep rubbing briskly, and at the same time, breathe deeply for one minute.

Next, place your hands at your waist with your thumbs on the ropelike muscles near the spine and your fingers wrapped around your sides. With your thumbs, apply firm, steady pressure in toward the spine on the outer edges of those ropy muscles, so that your thumbs are about four inches apart. This inward pressure stimulates B 47. You can also stimulate the inner point, B 23, by pressing the top of the large vertical muscles about two finger widths away from the spine. Use either your thumbs or your fingers to stimulate one side at a time or both sides at once, holding for at least one minute. Apply as much pressure as you can without causing discomfort.

Step 2

Knees to the chest: Lie on your back and inhale. Use your arms to pull your knees up to your chest and hold them with your arms as you exhale slowly. Then inhale, letting your knees come out, away from your chest. Repeat this movement for two minutes, breathing deeply into your diaphragm. As you use your arm muscles to bring your knees to your chest and exhale, feel your lower back flatten and stretch against the floor.

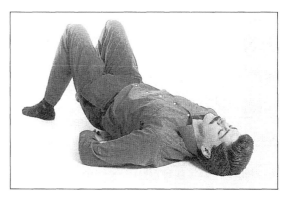

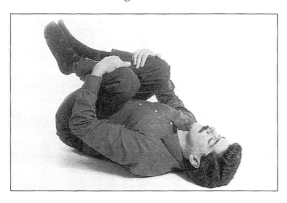

Relax after this exercise with your knees bent, feet flat on the floor, eyes closed, for at least three minutes. Practice twice a day.

Step 3

Firmly press CV 6: Place your fingertips in the lower abdominal area between your belly button and pubic bone. Gradually press one to two inches deep inside the abdomen as you breathe deeply for one minute.

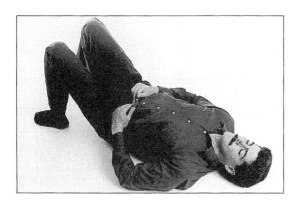

Step 4

Roll over the B 48 area: Place your hands underneath your buttocks (palms down) beside the base of the spine. Close your eyes and take long, deep breaths and rock your knees from side to side for two minutes. Reposition your hands for comfort and to enable different parts of the buttock muscles to be pressed. Also try swaying your legs from side to side with your knees pulled into your abdomen and your feet off the floor.

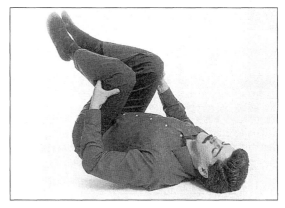

Step 5

Press B 54: Place your fingertips in the center of the crease behind your knees. Curving your fingers, use your arm muscles to rock your legs back and forth for one minute as you breathe deeply. Then let your feet rest flat on the floor, with knees bent, and relax.

Step 6

Press B 23 and B 47 again: Make fists and carefully place them on your lower back. Position your fists, palms facing down, so that the knuckles rest between your spine and your lower back muscles. Close your eyes and breathe deeply for one minute. Then slowly roll onto your side into a comfortable fetal position, with your arm under your head for a pillow. Close your eyes and relax deeply for at least five minutes.

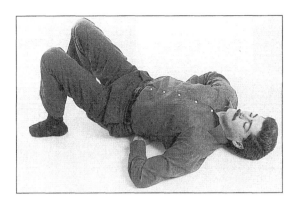

Tennis Ball Massage

Tennis balls can be helpful for applying acupressure on your lower back. Tightly roll up two balls close together in a large, thick towel or sock and place it on a carpeted floor. Sit down with the balls in back of you, your knees bent and feet flat on the floor. Lean back on your elbows, gradually reclining as the balls rest beneath your lower back.

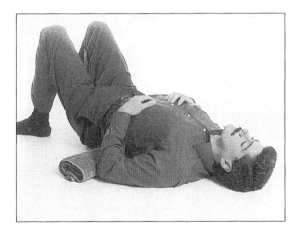

Take several long, slow, deep breaths. After a minute, gradually roll the balls onto another tense area. Hold that position for another minute while you take several more deep breaths with your eyes closed. Move them to another tense area.

After you have relieved most of your back tension, put the balls aside and lie down on your back. With your eyes closed, repeat step 2 for one minute. Then, completely relax for five minutes and continue deep breathing.

Additional Points for Relieving Lower-Back Aches and Sciatica

For illustrations of related points for relieving lower-back pain and sciatica, see chapter 33, "Neck Tension, Whiplash and Pain"; and chapter 35, "Pain."

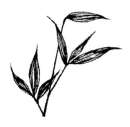

10

CHRONIC FATIGUE SYNDROME

$\mathcal{D}$escribed as the "malaise of the eighties" by *Newsweek* magazine, chronic fatigue syndrome's catalog of symptoms is growing as more data becomes available. It includes chronic fatigue, muscle pain and weakness, headaches, dizziness, nausea, depression, confused thinking, and irritability.

Chronic fatigue syndrome (Epstein-Barr) is widely believed to be a viral infection. The weakening of the immune system, which enables the virus to thrive, may occur as a result of exposure to environmental pollutants,[20] or as a consequence of severe stress.

Dr. Gerald Epstein observes, "In those individuals I've seen who were diagnosed as having Epstein-Barr virus it is clear that their life situations at the time of the occurrence had been somewhat overwhelming."[21]

According to traditional Chinese medicine, the health of the immune system is governed primarily by the condition of the kidney, liver, lungs, and spleen. The following routine uses points that fortify these organs to recharge the body and to strengthen its resistance to environmental and situational stresses. In addition, by fortifying the kidneys, acupressure awakens the body's self-curative abilities and strengthens the overall condition of the body.[22]

Jenny, a client of mine who tended to be generally weak and depressed, suffered from headaches and chronic fatigue syndrome. After briefly working on her shoulders and neck, I showed her how to use self-acupressure techniques to improve her condition: briskly rubbing the lower back, then the outsides of the legs below the knees, and finally the tops of the feet. Even though Jenny experienced a great sense of relaxation and revitalization after the one session, I advised her to work on the acupressure points at least three times a day. I told her that it would take several months of hard work and a lifetime of eating carefully to really help herself. Fortunately, Jenny is strong willed; she practices the self-acupressure every day and has been inspired with the results.

Each of the chronic fatigue syndrome relief points outlined below was chosen to deal with the primary symptoms of the condition as well as to strengthen the immune system and the body's resistance. Lu 1 improves the condition of the lungs. B 23 and B 47, in the lower back, benefit the kidneys, fortifying their vital energy to combat chronic fatigue. CV 6, in the lower abdominal area, promotes the optimal functioning of the internal organs. Pressing P 6, a famous trigger point located in the wrist, relieves nausea. GB 20, under the base of the skull, restores equilibrium to counteract dizziness. The Third Eye Point, between the eyebrows, is beneficial for clearing the mind of confusion. GB 21, on the top of the shoulder, relieves chronic shoulder tension and general stress.

All of the above potent points along with St 36, Lv 3, and TW 5 will fortify the body

---

[20] Robert A. Buist, Ph.D., "New Light on Chronic Fatigue Syndrome," *Health and Nutrition Update*, 4, no. 1 (1989).
[21] Gerald Epstein, M.D., *Creating Health Through Imagery* (New York: Bantam Books, 1989), 103.
[22] For more self-help techniques for relieving fatigue and a poor general condition, see Michael Reed Gach, *Acu-Yoga* (Tokyo: Japan Publications, 1981), 162-167.

with greater energy, awaken the immune system, and enable the internal organs to function at optimal levels. These chronic fatigue syndrome relief points are important to include in your overall treatment program for health maintenance and wellness.

Potent Points for Relieving Chronic Fatigue Syndrome (Epstein-Barr Virus)

Letting Go (Lu 1)

Location: On the outer part of the chest, four finger widths up from the armpit crease and one finger width inward.

Benefits: Relieves difficult breathing, fatigue, confusion, chest tension and congestion, emotional repression, coughing, and asthma.

Shoulder Well (GB 21)

Caution: Pregnant women should press this point *lightly*.

Location: On the highest point of the shoulder muscle, one to two inches from the side of the lower neck.

Benefits: Anxiety, irritability, fatigue, shoulder tension, poor circulation, cold hands or feet, nervous problems, and headaches.

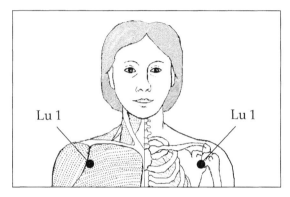

Gates of Consciousness (GB 20)

Location: Just below the base of the skull, in the hollow between the two large neck muscles, two to three inches apart depending on the size of the head.

Benefits: Relieves headaches, arthritis, insomnia, dizziness, stiff neck, neck pain, injuries, trauma, shock, hypertension, neuromotor coordination, eyestrain, and irritability.

Inner Gate (P 6)

Location: Two and one-half finger widths up the arm from the center of the inner wrist crease, midway between the two forearm bones.

Benefits: Relieves indigestion, nausea, insomnia, nervousness, palpitations, and wrist pain.

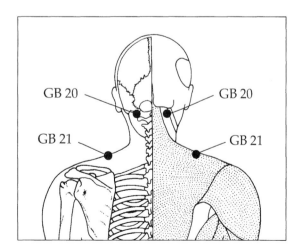

■ *You do not have to use all of these points. Using just one or two of them whenever you have a free hand can be effective.*

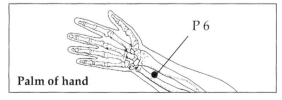

Outer Gate (TW 5)

Location: Two and one-half finger widths above the outer wrist crease, between the two forearm bones.

Benefits: Relieves rheumatism, tendonitis, wrist pain, and shoulder pain and increases resistance to colds and flus.

Sea of Vitality (B 23 and B 47)

Caution: Do not press on disintegrating discs or on fractured or broken bones. If you have a weak back, a few minutes of stationary, light touch instead of deep pressure can be very healing. See your doctor first if you have any questions or need medical advice.

Location: In the lower back two (B 23) and four (B 47) finger widths away from the spine at waist level.

Benefits: Relieves many chronic fatigue syndrome symptoms such as muscle weakness, extreme fatigue, irritability, dizziness, and confusion.

Three Mile Point (St 36)

Location: Four finger widths below the kneecap, one finger width on the outside of the shinbone. If you are on the correct spot, a muscle should flex as you move your foot up and down.

Benefits: Relieves fatigue, dizziness, and general weakness, as well as strengthens and tones the muscles throughout the body.

Bigger Rushing (Lv 3)

Location: On the top of the foot, in the valley between the big toe and the second toe.

Benefits: Relieves fainting, dizziness, fatigue, confusion, headaches, nausea, and irritability.

Third Eye Point (GV 24.5)

Location: Directly between the eyebrows, in the indentation where the bridge of the nose joins the forehead.

Benefits: Aids chronic fatigue syndrome complaints, especially irritability, confusion, and headaches.

Sea of Energy (CV 6)

Location: Three finger widths below the belly button.

Benefits: Relieves general weakness, extreme fatigue, dizziness, and confusion that results from the chronic fatigue syndrome.

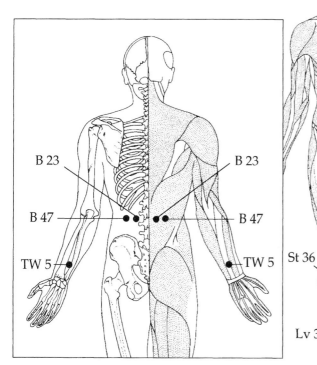

Potent Point Exercises

Lie down, or sit comfortably, and concentrate on breathing deeply as you hold each potent point. Deep abdominal breathing increases the circulation to every part of your body, washes away muscle stiffness, and infuses your body with vitality. The first three points relax the shoulders and strengthen the immune system.

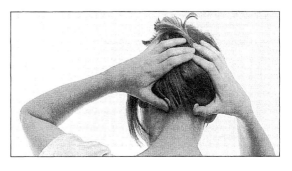

Step 3

Press up into GB 20: Place your thumbs underneath the base of your skull into the indentations between the two vertical neck muscles, two to three inches apart depending on the size of your head. Apply pressure gradually underneath the base of your skull as you slowly tilt your head back, and breathe deeply for one minute.

The next two points on your arms balance the immune system.

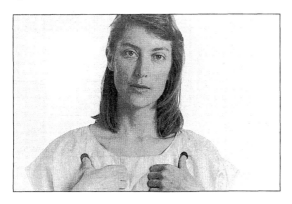

Step 1

Press Lu 1: Place your thumbs on the upper, outer portion of your chest and feel for a "knot" of tension. Make firm contact with the muscles located four finger widths up and one finger width inward from your armpit. Close your eyes and breathe deeply into your chest as you hold the point steadily for one minute.

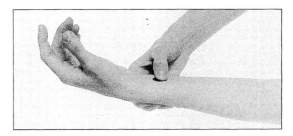

Step 4

Grasp P 6 and TW 5: Place your right thumb on the inside of your left wrist, two and one-half finger widths above the crease. Position your fingertips on the outside of your arm, directly behind your thumb on TW 5. Firmly grasp these points for thirty seconds, then switch wrists and hold the point for another thirty seconds.

Step 2

Firmly press GB 21: Curve your fingers on both hands, hooking them on the tops of your shoulders, where tension tends to collect. Close your eyes and breathe deeply for one minute as you imagine the healing energy flowing into your shoulders.

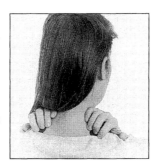

The following four steps of the potent point routine stimulate and fortify the immune system.

Step 5

Rub B 23 and B 47: Place the backs of your hands against your lower back. Briskly rub your knuckles in your lower back to create warmth for one minute. The vigorous rubbing in your lower back should be strenuous enough to get you out of breath. This stimulation will strengthen the immune system.

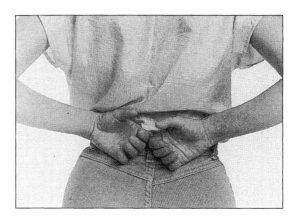

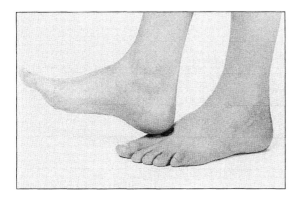

Step 7

Firmly rub Lv 3: Place your right heel on the top of your left foot at the junction between the bones that attach to your large and second toes. Use your heel to rub this important liver point for thirty seconds. Then switch sides, and rub the same point on your other foot.

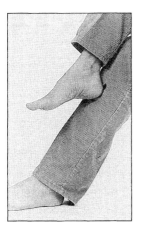

Step 6

Briskly rub St 36: Place the heel of your right foot on the St 36 point of your left leg a couple of inches below the kneecap and one finger width to the outside of the shinbone. Briskly rub it for one minute, then do the other side for another minute.

Step 8

Hold the GV 24.5 and CV 6: Use your right middle finger to lightly touch the Third Eye Point between your eyebrows. Place your left fingers in between your belly button and pubic bone to firmly press CV 6. Close your eyes and breathe deeply as you hold these points for two minutes.

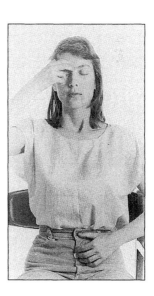

Additional Points for Relieving Chronic Fatigue Syndrome

For illustrations of related points for relieving chronic fatigue syndrome, see chapter 11, "Colds and Flu"; chapter 23, "Immune System Boosting"; and chapter 24, "Impotency and Sexual Problems."

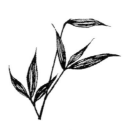

11

COLDS AND FLU

Colds are caused by viruses that thrive in your nose and throat when the temperature, acidity, and moisture suit them. When you are run down and your resistance is low, your ability to adapt to environmental changes weakens, making it easier to catch a cold, and the mucous membranes become a perfect breeding ground for viruses. Cold symptoms are the body's attempt to protect itself from these intruders. When a virus enters your nose, for instance, the body secretes more mucus to flush it away.

Because acupressure stimulates your body to expel the virus more quickly, it may seem at first that your cold is worsening. But your body is simply progressing through the symptoms faster than usual. Although acupressure cannot cure a cold, working on certain points can help you get better quicker and increase your resistance to future colds.

Seasonal Changes

Potent point B 36, called Bearing Support, is especially good for stimulating the body's natural resistance to colds and flus. It's located near the spine, off the tips of the shoulder blades. According to traditional Chinese medicine, wind and cold enter the pores of the skin at this point.[23] The muscles in this upper back area tend to get tense just before a cold or flu takes hold.[24]

Recently, one of my best friends, a realtor, was suffering from a bad cold with a stuffy nose, a hacking cough, puffiness around his eyes, and a pallid complexion. He hadn't slept well the previous two nights because of these discomforts and was very tired. After I briefly massaged his upper back, shoulders, neck, and chest, I showed him how to press the decongestion points underneath the base of his skull and on his face. I also told him to drink ginger tea at least twice a day. When I saw John the next day, he told me he had slept soundly and felt much more refreshed. His eyes looked much clearer, and already he was no longer coughing and blowing his nose.

B 36   B 36

---

[23] Felix Mann, *Treatment of Disease by Acupuncture* (London: William Heinemann Medical Books, Ltd., 1976), 32, 37.

[24] For more information and self-help techniques for colds and flu see Michael Reed Gach, *Acu-Yoga* (Tokyo: Japan Publications, 1981) pp. 138-142.

Potent Points for Relieving Colds and Flu

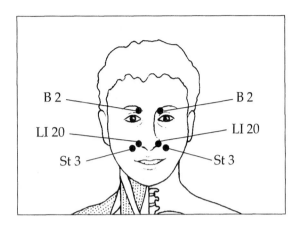

Drilling Bamboo (B 2)

Location: In the indentations of the eye sockets, on either side of where the bridge of the nose meets the ridge of the eyebrows.

Benefits: Relieves colds, sinus congestion, frontal headaches, and tired eyes.

Facial Beauty (St 3)

Location: At the bottom of the cheekbone, directly below the pupil.

Benefits: Relieves stuffy nose, head congestion, burning eyes, eye fatigue, and eye pressure.

Welcoming Perfume (LI 20)

Location: On either cheek, just outside each nostril.

Benefits: Relieves nasal congestion, sinus pain, facial paralysis, and facial swelling.

Crooked Pond (LI 11)

Location: At the outer end of the elbow crease.

Benefits: Relieves cold symptoms, fever, constipation, and elbow pain; strengthens the immune system.

Joining the Valley (Hoku) (LI 4)

Caution: This point is forbidden for pregnant women because its stimulation can cause premature contractions in the uterus.

Location: At the highest spot of the muscle on the back of the hand that protrudes when the thumb and index finger are close together.

Benefits: Relieves colds, flu, head congestion, constipation, and headaches.

Gates of Consciousness (GB 20)

Location: Below the base of the skull, in the hollows on both sides, two to three inches apart depending on the size of the head.

Benefits: Relieves headaches, head congestion, arthritis, neck pain, and irritability.

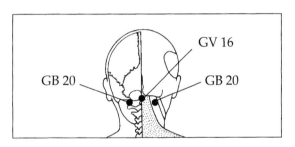

Wind Mansion (GV 16)

Location: In the center of the back of the head, in the large hollow under the base of the skull.

Benefits: Relieves head congestion, red eyes, mental stress, headaches, and stiff neck.

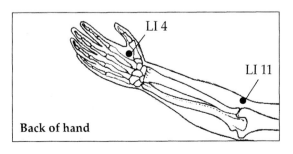

Back of hand

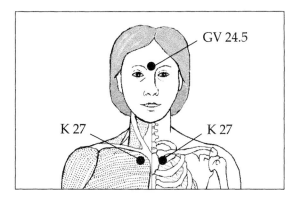

■ *You do not have to use all of these points. Using just one or two of them whenever you have a free hand can be effective.*

Third Eye Point (GV 24.5)

Location: Directly between the eyebrows, in the indentation where the bridge of the nose meets the center of your forehead.

Benefits: Relieves head congestion, stuffy nose, and headaches.

Elegant Mansion (K 27)

Location: In the hollow below the collarbone next to the breastbone.

Benefits: Relieves chest congestion, breathing difficulties, coughing, and sore throats.

Potent Point Exercises

Lie down on your back or sit comfortably.

Step 1

Press into B 2: Use your thumbs on the upper ridge of your eye socket to press into the slight hollow near the bridge of your nose for one minute. Close your eyes and take a few deep breaths, letting the weight of your head relax forward onto your thumbs.

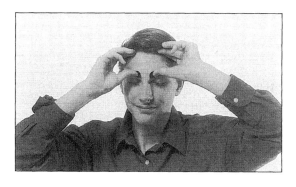

Step 2

Press St 3 and LI 20: Place both of your middle fingers beside your nostrils and your index fingers next to them; gradually press up and underneath the cheekbones for one minute. You can easily teach this step to your child to help relieve nasal congestion.

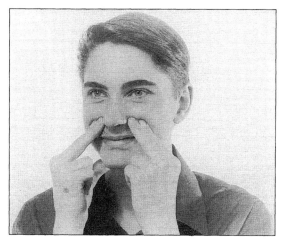

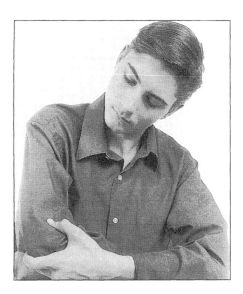

Step 3

Press both LI 11: Bend your arm and place your thumb at the end of the elbow crease on the outside of your forearm. Curve your fingers to press firmly into the elbow joint for one minute. Repeat on your opposite arm.

Step 4

Press LI 4 firmly: Spread your left thumb and index finger apart. Place your right thumb in the webbing on the back of your left hand and your fingertips on the palm directly behind

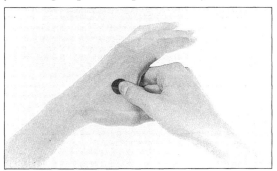

your thumb. Firmly squeeze your thumb and index finger of your right hand together to press into the webbing. Angle the pressure toward the bone that connects with your left index finger, and hold for one minute. Then switch hands.

Step 5

Firmly press GB 20: Now close your eyes and place your thumbs underneath the base of your skull, two to three inches apart. Slowly tilt your head back and apply pressure gradually, holding the position for one minute to fully release these important cold-relief points.

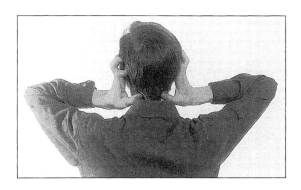

Step 6

Firmly press GV 16: Place the tips of your middle fingers into the hollow in the center of the base of your skull. Keeping your fingers on the point, inhale as you tilt your head back and exhale as you relax your head forward. Continue to slowly rock your head back and forward, and breathe deeply while you hold this important point for relieving head congestion.

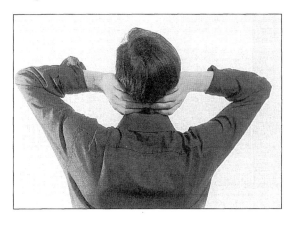

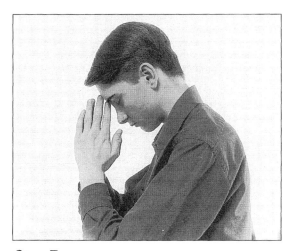

Step 7
Touch the GV 24.5: Bring your palms together and use your middle and index fingers to lightly touch the Third Eye Point located between your eyebrows. Breathe deeply as you hold this point for balancing your endocrine system.

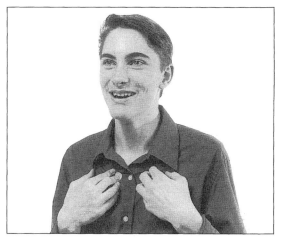

Step 8
Firmly press K 27: Place your fingertips on the protrusions of your collarbone, then slide your fingers down and outward into the first indentation in between the bones. Press into this hollow as you breathe deeply and visualize the congestion clearing.

Potent Points for Relieving Coughing

A severe, repeated, or uncontrolled cough can be harmful and you should always consult a physician. Many illnesses such as influenza, pneumonia, and chronic bronchitis can become serious if the condition continues unattended.

Sometimes, your physician will find it advisable to attempt to suppress a cough to prevent further irritation of the bronchial tubes. Cough medications may be used, but acupressure can be an effective adjunct therapy. During a coughing fit, many of the large muscle groups in the upper back area can go into a spasm. Specific points on the chest, throat, neck, and upper back benefit the respiratory system, relax your body, and relieve coughs.

Vital Diaphragm (B 38)
Location: Between the shoulder blade and the spine at the level of the heart.

Benefits: Relieves coughing, breathing difficulties, and respiratory problems. This calming point also helps balance the emotions.

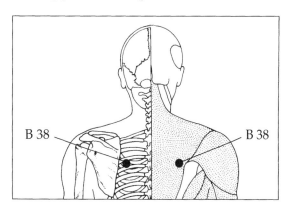

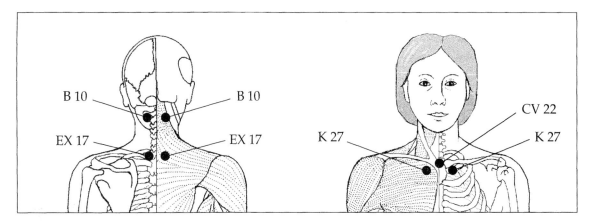

Ding Chuan (Extra Point 17)

Location: To the side and a little above the vertebra that protrudes at the top of the spine when the head is tilted downward.

Benefits: Relieves throat problems, coughing, shoulder and neck pain, and thyroid imbalances.

Heavenly Pillar (B 10)

Location: One-half inch below the base of the skull on the ropy muscles one-half inch out from either side of the spine.

Benefits: Relieves sore throat, stress, burnout, overexertion, and heaviness in the head.

Heaven Rushing Out (CV 22)

Location: At the base of the throat in the large hollow directly below the Adam's apple.

Benefits: Relieves dry cough, bronchitis, sore throat, chest congestion, and heartburn.

Elegant Mansion (K 27)

Location: In the hollow below the collarbone next to the breastbone.

Benefits: Relieves chest congestion, breathing difficulties, asthma, coughing, and anxiety.

■ *You do not have to use all of these points. Using just one or two of them whenever you have a cough can be effective.*

Potent Point Exercises

Although many of the following points can be held while you are sitting, it is preferable to lie down comfortably on your back.

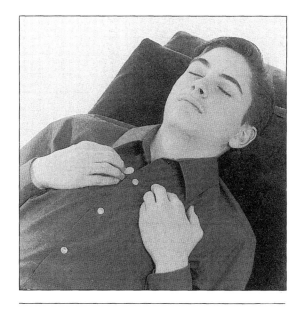

Step 1

Hold both K 27 points: Place your fingertips on your chest and firmly press into the indentations directly below the protrusions of the collarbone. This is another point that you can easily teach a child.

Step 2

Use tennis balls[25] on B 38: Place two small rubber balls or tennis balls together on a clean carpet. Lie down, placing the balls between your shoulder blades at the level of your heart. Close your eyes and take three long, deep breaths as you continue to press the K 27 points on your upper chest.

[25] This step is optional. If you don't have tennis balls or a pair of small rubber balls, feel free to skip this point.

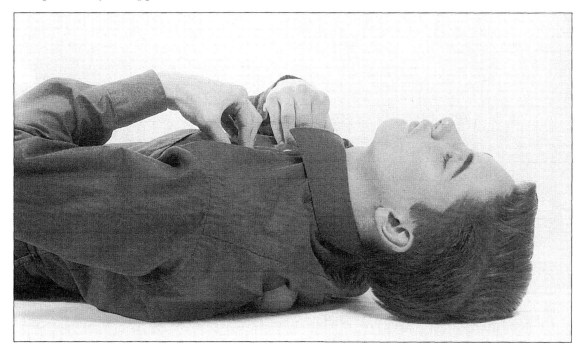

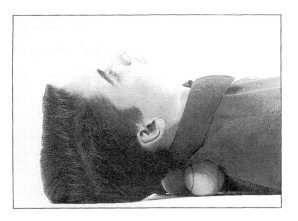

Step 3

Firmly press extra point 17: Slowly roll the tennis balls a few inches higher toward the base of your neck. If the tennis balls tend to slip, or you aren't using them, simply use both middle fingers to press this important acupressure point at the base of the neck.

Step 4

Hold both B 10 points and CV 22: Press B 10 on the upper neck with one hand, using the fingertips. Use your other hand to lightly hold

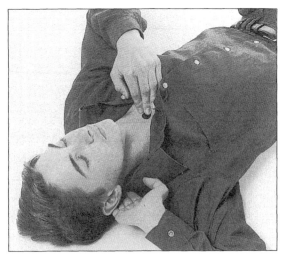

CV 22, an inch below the base of the Adam's apple, pressing lightly at a downward angle. Close your eyes and breathe deeply as you visualize healing energy soothing your throat.

For Sore Throats and Coughing

A small piece of fresh ginger can be one of the most natural and effective ways for soothing a sore throat. Simply place a very thin slice of fresh ginger on the back of your tongue. If your throat is sensitive and the ginger feels hot, use a smaller, thinner piece and place it farther back toward your throat. Keep the ginger in the back of your throat for ten minutes. Repeat with a fresh piece several times a day as needed. A quarter cup of chopped ginger can also be simmered in a few cups of water and used as a tea for soothing coughs and sore throats.

Additional Points for Relieving Colds and Flu

For illustrations of related points for relieving colds and flu, see chapter 8, "Asthma and Breathing Difficulties"; chapter 20, "Headaches and Migraines"; and chapter 38, "Sinus Problems and Hay Fever."

12
CONSTIPATION

One of my past clients who had numerous surgeries, including two cesareans and lower back surgery, was unable to have a bowel movement without tremendous pain. I showed her how to apply acupressure to her abdominal area (CV 6). Pressing this point encourages peristalsis and relaxes the abdomen. Within one month, after working on herself twice a day, she was able to have regular, painless bowel movements.

Constipation can be caused by eating too many refined, processed foods, such as white flour, that do not supply us with enough roughage; rich or heavy foods; too many different kinds of foods at once;[26] abdominal tension; or lack of exercise. Any one of these conditions can cause matter to block the colon. Constipation is often accompanied by gas, abdominal pain, bloating, and headaches, caused by the lack of peristaltic movement, which impels waste through the colon. The colon muscle can become too relaxed, too tired, or too tense to move.

Health experts agree that you can prevent constipation by eating properly and getting enough exercise. Whole foods such as fresh fruits and vegetables and whole grains contain roughage that encourages proper elimination of waste. A salad made from fresh spinach, parsley, lettuce, cucumbers, sprouts, bell peppers, and green beans is high in fiber and vitamins A, B, C, E, G, and K, all of which help relieve constipation.[27]

Exercises such as brisk walking, jogging, swimming, and Acu-Yoga[28] tone and massage the muscles of the intestinal tract, promote regularity of the bowels, and keep your whole body energized.

---

[26] Please see chapter 39, Stomachaches, Indigestion, and Heartburn, for a discussion of food combining.

[27] Mildred Jackson, N.D., *The Handbook of Alternatives to Chemical Medicine* (Oakland: Lawton-Teague Publications, 1975), p. 52.

[28] For more information, see Michael Reed Gach, *Acu-Yoga* (Tokyo: Japan Publications, 1981) pp. 142-147, 184-189.

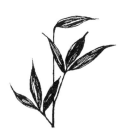

Potent Points for Relieving Constipation

Sea of Energy (CV 6)

Location: Three finger widths directly below the belly button.

Benefits: Relieves pain in the abdominal muscles, constipation, colitis, and gas.

Three Mile Point (St 36)

Location: Four finger widths below the kneecap, one finger width to the outside of the shinbone. If you are on the correct spot, a muscle should flex as you move your foot up and down.

Benefits: Strengthens the whole body, aids digestion, and relieves stomach and intestinal disorders.

Joining the Valley (Hoku) (LI 4)

Caution: This point is forbidden for pregnant women, because its stimulation can cause premature contractions in the uterus.

Location: At the highest spot of the muscle on the back of the hand that protrudes when the thumb and index finger are brought close together.

Benefits: Relieves constipation, headaches, toothaches, shoulder pain, arthritis, and labor pain.

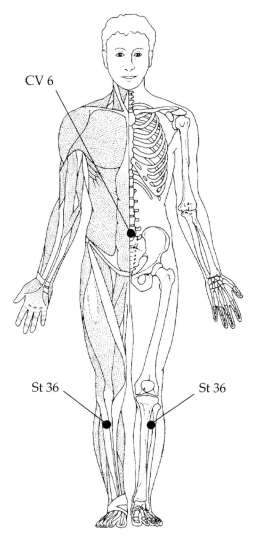

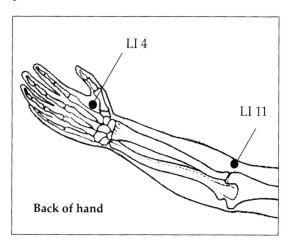

Back of hand

Crooked Pond (LI 11)

Location: At the outer end of the elbow crease.

Benefits: Relieves fever, constipation, and indigestion. This is a powerful trigger point for the colon.

■ *You do not have to use all of these points. Using just one or two of them whenever you have a free hand can be effective.*

Potent Point Exercises

For best results, start this routine lying down on your back.

Step 1

Firmly press CV 6: Place all of your fingertips directly between your navel and pubic bone. Gradually press in one inch deep or until you can lightly touch something firm. Maintain this firm pressure while you breathe deeply and keep your eyes closed.

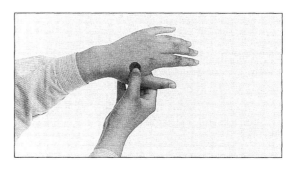

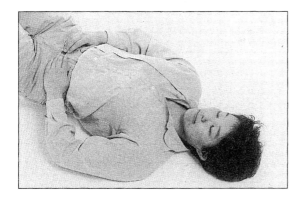

Step 3

Firmly squeeze LI 4: Spread your left thumb and index finger apart. Place your right thumb in the webbing in the back of your left hand and your fingertips on the palm directly behind your thumb. Gradually squeeze the thumb and index finger of your right hand together to firmly press into the webbing. Angle the pressure in toward the bone that connects with your left index finger. Take three long, slow, deep breaths as you continue to press the webbing of your left hand for one minute. Now switch sides and press LI 4 on your right hand. Press the webbing firmly as you take another few long, slow, deep breaths.

Step 2

Stimulate St 36: Place your right heel on the outside of the left shinbone beneath your knee. Briskly rub this point for one minute. Then do the same on the opposite leg.

Step 4

Press point LI 11: Bend your right arm in front of you with your palm facing down. To find this point place the fingertips of your left hand on the outside of your right forearm,

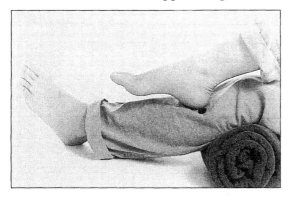

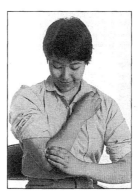

where the elbow crease ends. Breathe deeply as you firmly press into this point for one minute. Now switch hands and massage LI 11 on your other arm. Breathe deeply as you firmly press this point in the elbow joint for one minute.

Acupressure Massage

This routine further decongests the body and improves the resiliency and tone of the large intestine. It can be done either on another person or on oneself. The following are instructions for working on yourself. For obvious reasons, practice this routine on an empty stomach.

1. Lie down comfortably on your back, with knees up, feet flat on the floor, and your eyes closed.
2. Starting at the top of the abdomen, use all your fingertips to gradually press into the acupressure points located on the abdomen in a circle the size of your hand (see photograph). Press in slowly and hold each position for five seconds each, moving in a clockwise direction.
3. Breathe deeply as you repeat the slow clockwise rotation on the abdominal points, pressing a little more firmly the second and third times around.
4. Place your hands by your sides and completely relax as you continue to breathe deeply to assimilate the benefits.

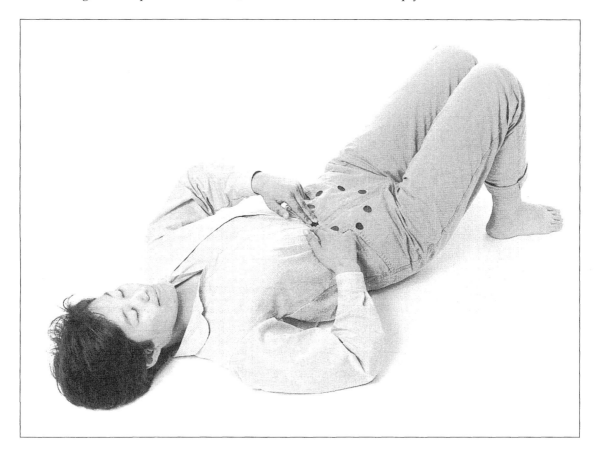

Additional Points for Relieving Constipation

For illustrations of other related points for relieving constipation, see chapter 15, "Diarrhea"; chapter 26, "Irritability, Frustration, and Dealing with Change"; and chapter 39, "Stomachaches, Indigestion, and Heartburn."

13
CRAMPS AND SPASMS

$\mathcal{B}$arbara, a friend of mine in her mid-forties, often suffered from foot cramps. When the toes of her feet would go into a spasm, it became almost impossible for her to walk. As a nurse, she is required to be on her feet all day. In the past, she had taken pain pills for the cramps. After ten minutes of holding the three points on her ankles and feet described in the next exercise, her cramping and pain subsided.

The first time I showed her the points we were both surprised at how quickly a very painful and long-standing problem yielded to a few minutes of acupressure. Barbara now uses these points on herself almost every day and has been able to decrease the number of spasms dramatically.

Cramps are usually caused or worsened by muscular tension. During a cramp the nerves of the affected muscle are hyperactive, causing an extreme and sudden contraction of the muscle, the cramp, or spasm. Tense muscles already in a contracted state inhibit circulation so that lactic acid and other toxins accumulate. This buildup further imbalances the area and increases muscle tension.

Cramps can develop in any muscle in the body, but they usually occur in muscles that have been overused. Runners, for instance, tend to get cramps in their feet or legs. Also, muscles used a great deal at one time may develop cramps years later if muscle tone is not maintained.

If you get a leg cramp while running and relieve it with acupressure, do not run for the rest of the day. When you've completely released the cramp, walk gently to rebalance your leg muscles.

Acupressure Points

Acupressure points help relieve muscle cramps in two ways: by using a specific point associated with cramps and by pressing points directly on the cramped muscle.

The first method uses both the antispasmodic trigger point GV 26 and point Lv 3 to prevent cramps and spasms. Lv 3 is located on the top of the foot in the valley between the large and second toes. If you get a cramp, immediately press GV 26 strongly. Prolonged firm pressure on this point quickly releases the cramp. This is something you can easily teach your child.

The second method uses a point in the affected area to release a cramped muscle. This direct method involves pressing very gradually into the heart of the cramped muscle and maintaining the pressure for about two or three minutes. This prolonged pressure counters the force of the cramp. As long as you hold the point with steady, firm pressure, you can outlast the force of the cramp, and the muscle spasm will yield to your pressure and simply relax. After the cramp has eased, hold Lv 3 and the local point gently for a few more minutes to balance the area.

Diet

Certain foods are associated with cramps. Foods that tend to constrict and tighten the muscles lay a foundation for potential cramping problems. Meats and salt are foods that have a contracting effect on the muscles. When eaten in excess, these foods contribute to tension: Salt causes water retention and

meat, when eaten in excess, can cause constipation. Traditional Oriental health care
teaches that excess salt tends to stiffen the
muscles and has an overall rigidifying effect.

Cramps can also be caused by a calcium
deficiency. Vitamins D and E assist in the
assimilation of calcium, and it's important to
get enough of them. Fresh lemon juice in a
glass of warm water, for example, provides
the body with these vitamins.[29]

In traditional Chinese medicine, muscle
cramps are related to the liver. The food
flavor associated with the liver is sourness.
A moderate amount of sour-flavored foods in
one's diet improves muscle tone and aids in
preventing cramps. Conversely, an excess
amount of sour or salty foods can cause
rigidity and stiffness in muscles.[30]

Preventing Cramps

Prevention is the best solution for cramps.
Both Acu-Yoga[31] stretches, which use yoga
postures to press the points, and acupressure
massage help keep the muscles flexible, which
is the surest way to prevent cramping.

Acu-Yoga helps in two ways. First, it
increases your awareness of muscle tension, so
that you know which areas of your body need
the most attention. Second, the yoga postures
gently stretch, loosen, and relax the muscles,
thereby easing the tension that prompts
cramping and spasms.

Massaging tense muscles that tend to
cramp up is also helpful. If you have a
problem with cramps in a particular area,
daily massage and the occasional use of hot
compresses help relax muscular tension. For
example, if your calf muscles tend to cramp,
knead the entire length of the muscle. Be sure
to apply pressure to potent point B 57 (described on the next page) as well as massage
the area from the Achilles tendon, above the
heel, to the back of the knee. Whenever a
muscle feels particularly tense, take fifteen to
twenty minutes for massage and stretching,
and apply heat to loosen it up before it gets to
the point of cramping.

The following acupressure points help
tone and relax the muscles to prevent cramps
and spasms.

[29] Mildred Jackson, N.D., *The Handbook of Alternatives to Chemical Medicine* (Oakland: Lawton-Teague Publications, 1975), 68.
[30] Ilza Veith, *The Yellow Emperor's Classic of Internal Medicine* (Berkeley: University of California Press) 21-23.
[31] See Michael Reed Gach, *Acu-Yoga: Self-Help Techniques to Relieving Tension* (Tokyo: Japan Publications, 1981), 148-151.

Potent Points for Relieving Cramps and Spasms

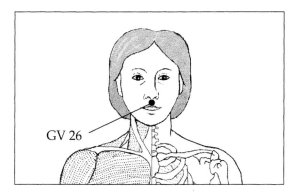

Middle of a Person (GV 26)

Location: Two-thirds of the way up from the upper lip to the nose.

Benefits: This first-aid revival point has traditionally been used for cramps, fainting, and dizziness.

Supporting Mountain (B 57)

For a leg cramp in the calf, focus on the following acupressure point.

Location: In the center of the base of the calf muscle, midway between the crease behind the knee and the heel, at the bottom of the calf muscle bulge.

Benefits: Relieves leg cramps (especially in the calf muscle), knee pain, lumbago, and feet swelling.

Bigger Rushing (Lv 3)

Location: On the top of the foot in the valley between the big toe and the second toe.

Benefits: Relieves foot cramps, headaches, tired eyes, and hangovers, as well as allergies and arthritis.

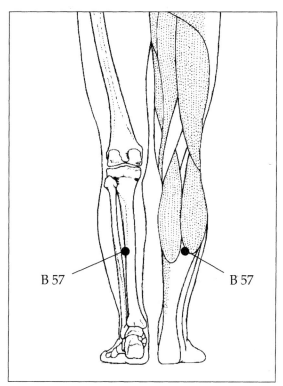

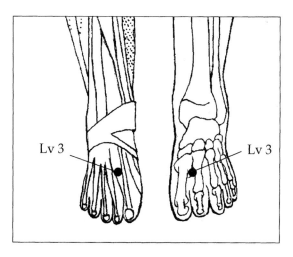

■ *You do not have to use all of these points. Using just one or two of them whenever you have a free hand can be effective.*

Potent Point Exercises

Sit comfortably for the following short routine.

Step 1

Firmly press GV 26: Use your index finger or a knuckle to apply enough pressure between your nose and upper lip to stimulate this antispasmodic point in your gum. Hold for one minute as you breathe deeply.

Step 2

Apply pressure to B 57: Use your thumbs to press the center of the base of your calf muscles. This point is typically very sensitive; therefore, carefully apply gradual pressure. Hold these muscle-relaxant points for one full minute.

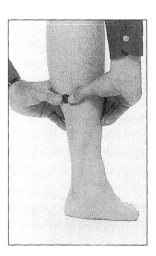

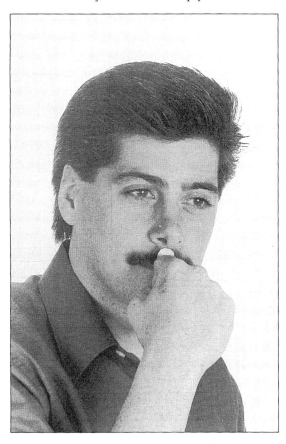

Step 3

Stimulate Lv 3: Place your index and middle fingers on the top of your feet into the hollow

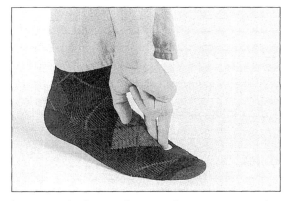

between the bones that attach to your second and big toes. Firmly rub and angle your pressure toward the bone of your second toe for one minute.

Additional Points for Relieving Cramps and Spasms

For illustrations of related points for relieving cramps and spasms, see chapter 5, "Ankle and Foot Problems"; chapter 28, "Knee Pain"; and chapter 35, "Pain."

14
DEPRESSION AND EMOTIONAL BALANCING

*D*epression is an emotional disorder characterized by sadness, inactivity, grief, difficulty concentrating, feelings of loss, or emotional withdrawal. Depression can be a signal that something in our life may be lacking or out of balance. We often get depressed, for example, when we lack a sense of purpose to our lives or when we lack close, nurturing relationships. Depression can become a vicious circle of cause and effect that often leads to self-defeating behavior, which in turn further deepens the depression. As our morale and self-esteem suffer, we "shut down," both emotionally and physically.

It is important to distinguish between a short-term, run-of-the-mill depression — what you might call the "blues" — and a more chronic, acute depression. For the latter, professional counseling or therapy are necessary. However, the acupressure and deep relaxation techniques described in this chapter are extremely beneficial self-help treatments for a mild depression or emotional funk.

Depression can also result from repressed emotions and energies. The antidepression points in this chapter release energies inside us that have been blocked. As you release the points, the blocked parts of the body open up, and the feelings repressed by that blockage can surface. You may then be able to gain a new awareness of these feelings and battle the roots of your depression.

Lifestyle

The following four concepts help develop personal fulfillment, which is important for preventing depression.
- *Self-Love:* Decide to create or cultivate positive situations that fulfill your personal needs, encourage growth, and promote self-esteem.
- *Mutual Relationships:* Become involved with people who have a positive attitude, who share in giving and receiving, and who show their love.
- *Meaningful Work:* Find a form of service that contributes to your sense of purpose and identity.
- *Goals and Visions for the Future:* Visualize desirable changes in your life and make goals for working toward them.

Diet

Depression can also result from hypoglycemia (low blood sugar), a condition characterized by fluctuating emotions from extreme highs to extreme lows. Hypoglycemia can be caused by too much sugar in the diet. For the short-term, the consumption of sugar raises the blood sugar level producing a sudden burst of energy. To balance this extreme surge of blood sugar, however, the pancreas then overproduces insulin, which drastically lowers the blood sugar level, causing fatigue, depression, and anxiety.

Sufferers of hypoglycemia should avoid sugar, alcohol, coffee, and fruits with a high sugar content. Fresh vegetables, whole grains, miso soup, sprouts, and seaweed are excellent foods that balance the above substances.

Depression can also be caused by deficiencies of vitamins C and E. Salads of parsley and cucumber dressed with fresh lemon juice, for example, are a rich source of these vitamins.

An emotional imbalance can also result from shallow breathing that causes an inadequate supply of oxygen in the blood. You can remedy this deficiency in two ways: First, by pressing the potent points described in this chapter to increase blood circulation; and second, with deep breathing, which increases the oxygen supply and enhances the benefits of acupressure.

Notice your breathing when you are feeling low; it tends to be shallow and constricted. A simple, effective technique for combating mild depression is to increase the depth of your breathing. This sounds simple, but it requires deep concentration. Close your eyes and focus your full attention on breathing deeply. This relaxes your body and will naturally open your mind to experience positive thoughts and creative images. If you increase the depth of your breath so that you are taking no more than four breaths a minute, within five minutes this exercise will change the way you feel. Try it.

Quick Tips for Relieving Depression

After practicing just two of the following tips, your depression may go away!

- **Aerobic Exercise:** Just twenty to thirty minutes of bicycling, swimming, dancing (just put some good music on and move it!), running, or brisk walking can relieve most common, mild depressions.
- **Take a Stimulating Shower:** Start showering with warm water, gradually making it hotter. Then decrease the temperature as low as you can stand it. Cold water stimulates the nerves close to the surface of the skin and is rejuvenating. *Do not do this if you have a serious illness (see the caution on page 9) or are pregnant, premenstrual, or menstruating.*
- **Deep Breathing Exercises:** In just ten minutes, you can oxygenate your body and relieve your depression by practicing deep breathing and relaxation.
- **Movement and Breathing Meditation:** In just five minutes the following acupressure breathing exercise, "Letting Go of Depression," will deepen your breathing and enable you to feel better and in control.

Letting Go of Depression

1. Lie down on your back or sit comfortably, with your spine straight, and feet flat on the floor.

2. Reach up toward the sky with both hands; take a deep breath, and as you hold your breath, make tight fists and squeeze, tightening all the muscles in your arms.

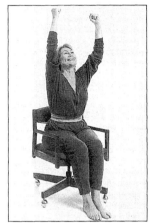

3. Slowly exhale, tensing your arms, bringing your fists down to your chest.

4. Repeat steps 2 and 3 several times.

5. Now cross your arms in front of your chest, with your fingers touching the upper outside area of the chest, which will probably be tight (Lu 1); your wrists cross at the center of your upper chest.

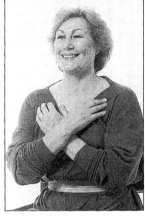

6. Lower your chin toward your chest.

7. Inhale four short breaths in a row (without exhaling) through your nose, filling your lungs completely on the fourth breath. Hold the breath for a few seconds with the chest full and expanded.

8. Exhale slowly through your mouth.

9. Repeat this exercise for two or three minutes, concentrating on the depth and rhythm of the breath.

Potent Points for Relieving Depression

Vital Diaphragm (B 38)

Location: Between the shoulder blades and the spine at the level of the heart.

Benefits: This calming point helps to balance the emotions. It relieves anxiety, grief, and other emotional imbalances.

Heavenly Pillar (B 10)

Location: One-half inch below the base of the skull, on the ropy muscles located one-half inch out from the spine.

Benefits: Relieves emotional distress, burn-out, exhaustion, depression, and heaviness in the head.

Gates of Consciousness (GB 20)

Location: Below the base of the skull, in the hollows between two large neck muscles, two to three inches apart depending on the size of the head.

Benefits: Relieves depression, headaches, dizziness, stiff necks, and irritability.

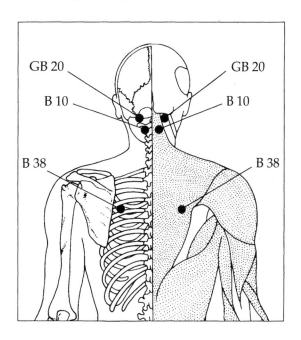

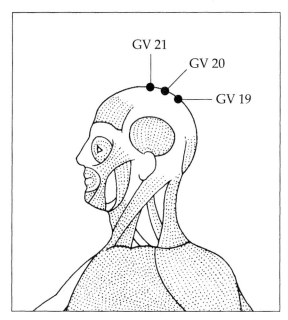

The following three antidepressant points are located on the top of the head.

Posterior Summit (GV19)
One Hundred Meeting Point (GV 20)
Anterior Summit (GV 21)

Locations: Start at GV 20, by placing the left fingers behind the left ear; the right fingers behind the right ear. Move the fingertips up to the top of the head, then feel for the hollow (GV 20) toward the back of the top, center of the head. GV 19 is also in a hollow, one inch in back of GV 20. GV 21 is one inch in front of GV 20.

Benefits: Relieves depression, headaches, and vertigo, and improves memory.

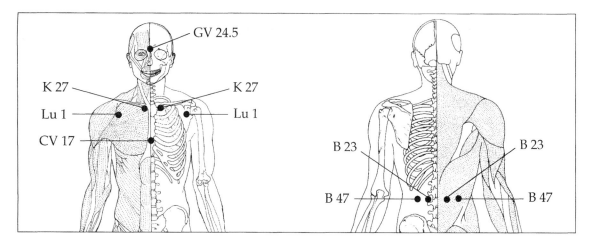

Elegant Mansion (K 27)

Location: In the indentation between the first rib and the lower border of the collarbone, just outside the upper breastbone.

Benefits: Relieves anxiety, depression, chest congestion, breathing difficulties, asthma, coughing, sore throats, and premenstrual tension.

Letting Go (Lu 1)

Location: On the outer part of the upper chest, four finger widths up from the armpit crease and one finger width inward.

Benefits: Relieves depression, grief, repressed emotions, shallow breathing, chest tension or congestion, coughing, asthma, and skin disorders.

Sea of Vitality (B 23 and B 47)

Caution: Do not press on disintegrating discs or a fractured or broken bone. If your back is in a weak condition, lightly touch these points, keeping your fingers stationary and exerting no pressure. See your doctor first if you have any questions or need medical advice.

Location: In the lower back two (B 23) and four (B 47) finger widths from the spine at waist level.

Benefits: Relieves depression, fatigue, exhaustion, trauma, and fear.

Third Eye Point (GV 24.5)

Location: Directly between the eyebrows in the indentation where the bridge of the nose meets the center of the forehead.

Benefits: Relieves depression as well as glandular and emotional imbalances.

Sea of Tranquility (CV 17)

Location: On the center of the breastbone three thumb widths up from the base of the bone.

Benefits: Relieves nervousness, chest congestion, grief, depression, hysteria, and other emotional imbalances.

Three Mile Point (St 36)

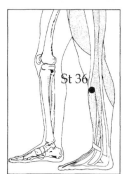

Location: Four finger widths below the kneecap, one finger width on the outside of the shinbone.

Benefits: Strengthens the whole body, tones the muscles, balances the emotions, and relieves fatigue, and counteracts depression.

■ *You do not have to use all of these points. Using just one or two of them whenever you have a free hand can be effective.*

Potent Point Exercises

Practice the first four steps of this routine lying down. Concentrate on breathing slowly and deeply throughout all of these self-acupressure massage techniques. Deep breathing increases circulation to every part of your body, washes away tension, relieves depression, and infuses your body with vitality.

Step 1

Use tennis balls to press B 38: Lie down on your back, placing two tennis balls on the floor underneath your upper back between your shoulder blades. (If the pressure from the balls hurts, place a thick towel, folded in half, over the tennis balls.) Then close your eyes, and breathe long and deep for two minutes.

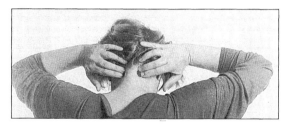

Step 2

Firmly press B 10 and GB 20: Use your fingertips to firmly press B 10 on both sides of the ropy muscles on your neck for one minute. Then use your thumbs to gradually press up underneath the skull into GB 20 as you slowly tilt your head back and breathe deeply for another minute.

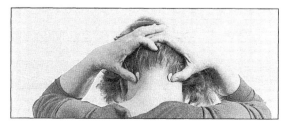

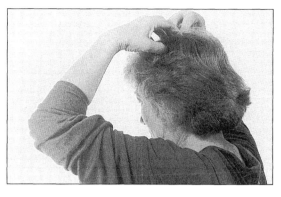

Step 3

Stimulate GV 19, GV 20, and GV 21: Place your fingertips on the center on the top of your head, then briskly rub with all your fingertips to stimulate these antidepressant points for one minute.

Step 4

Firmly press K 27 and Lu 1: Use your fingertips on both sides of your chest to firmly press K 27 and then Lu 1 for one minute each.

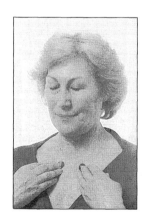

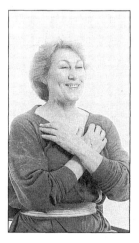

Slowly sit up and continue.

Step 5

Briskly rub B 23 and B 47: Make fists and place your knuckles against your lower back, two inches apart on either side of your spine. Briskly rub your back up and down for one minute to create heat.

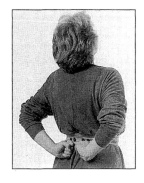

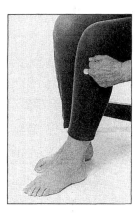

Step 6

Stimulate St 36: Place your left fist on St 36 of your left leg and briskly rub it for one minute. Then do the same on the other side.

Step 7

Third Eye Visualization: Sitting with your spine straight, eyes closed, chin tilted down slightly, bring your palms together and use your middle and index fingertips to lightly touch the Third Eye Point. Take long, slow,

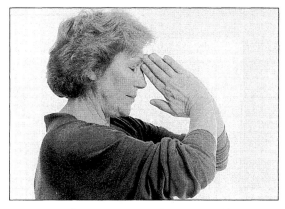

deep breaths as you visualize yourself going to a place that makes you feel calm, restful, and safe — a place where you can trust yourself to follow whatever steps you need to take to reach fulfillment in your life.

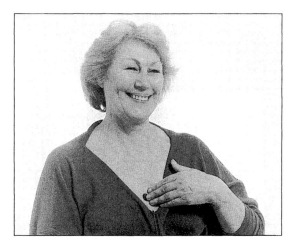

Step 8

Press CV 17: Use all of the fingertips of one hand to gently press the center of your breastbone as you take several more long, slow, deep breaths to enhance the benefits.

Additional Points for Relieving Depression

For illustrations of other related points for relieving depression, see chapter 6, "Anxiety and Nervousness"; chapter 8, "Asthma and Breathing Difficulties"; and chapter 10, "Chronic Fatigue Syndrome."

15
DIARRHEA

*A*cupressure can tone the abdominal region and balance the digestive system to relieve diarrhea. The points in the stomach area can directly affect the condition of the intestines. Finger pressure in this region is used like a pump, exercising the abdominal muscles and digestive organs. Acupressure points on the legs and feet also trigger signals to the digestive system to stop diarrhea. If you have severe diarrhea, be certain to call your doctor. Children who have diarrhea should be treated gently with acupressure only after diagnosis and approval by a pediatrician.

The abdominal points Sp 16 and CV 6 tone the abdominal area; potent points St 36, Sp 4, and Lv 2 on the legs and feet rebalance the gastrointestinal system by means of a triggering mechanism that stimulates the absorption of water in the intestines. By pressing these points three to four times a day, you can rebalance your internal organs to function harmoniously and alleviate diarrhea.

Diet: A diet for relieving diarrhea should be high in protein and carbohydrates, but low in fiber. Avoid cold, sweet foods (ice cream, soda, and sugar), and limit your intake of fruits and juices. A one-day fast can also help relieve diarrhea, but regularly drink a moderate amount of water or tea to prevent dehydration — a real danger with diarrhea. Consult your doctor before fasting. Try simmering one teaspoon of ginger root (preferably fresh ginger) in one cup of boiling water. Drinking this ginger tea three times daily helps relieve diarrhea.

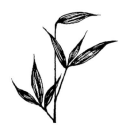

Potent Points for Relieving Diarrhea

Abdominal Sorrow (Sp 16)

Location: Below the edge of the rib cage one-half inch in from the nipple line.

Benefits: Relieves diarrhea, ulcer pain, indigestion, appetite imbalances, and abdominal cramps.

Sea of Energy (CV 6)

Location: Two finger widths directly below the belly button.

Benefits: Relieves chronic diarrhea, constipation, and gas; strengthens the abdominal muscles.

Three Mile Point (St 36)

Location: Four finger widths below the kneecap, one finger width on the outside of the shinbone. If you are on the correct spot, a muscle should flex as you move your foot up and down.

Benefits: Strengthens the whole body, tones the muscles, aids digestion, and relieves stomach disorders.

Grandfather Grandson (Sp 4)

Location: On the arch of the foot, one thumb width in back of the ball of the foot.

Benefits: Relieves indigestion, diarrhea, stomachaches, and nausea.

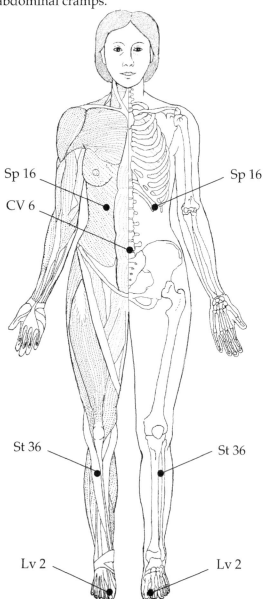

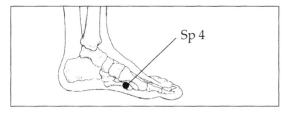

Travel Between (Lv 2)

Location: At the juncture of the big and second toes.

Benefits: Relieves diarrhea, stomachaches, headaches, and nausea.

■ *You do not have to use all of these points. Using just one or two of them whenever you have a free hand can be effective.*

Potent Point Exercises

Lie down on your back or sit in a comfortable position.

Step 1

Hold both Sp 16 points: Curve your fingers, placing your fingertips underneath the base of the ribs directly below the nipple line. Hold the indentations at the base of your rib cage while you breathe deeply for one minute to rebalance the gastrointestinal system.

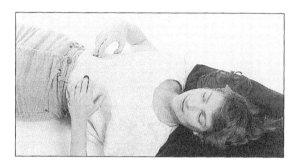

Step 2

Firmly press CV 6: Place all of your fingertips directly between your belly button and the center of your pubic bone. Gradually increase the depth of pressure in your lower abdomen. Close your eyes and breathe deeply as you press CV 6 for two minutes to balance and tone the colon.

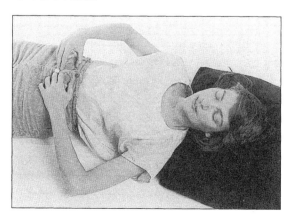

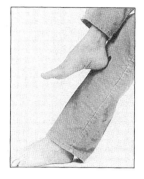

Step 3

Briskly rub St 36: Place your right heel on St 36 on your left leg and briskly rub it for one minute. Then stimulate the other side for one minute.

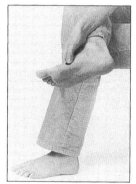

Step 4

Grasp Sp 4: Bend your right leg, placing your right foot on your left knee. Use your right thumb to press Sp 4 on the arch of your right foot. Hold firmly for a minute, Then switch sides.

Step 5

Hold Lv 2 on both sides: Press into the webbing between your big and second toes, angling your pressure toward the base of your big toe. Press firmly as you take three long, deep breaths.

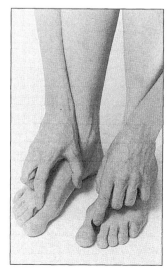

Step 6

Restimulate St 36: Use your heel again to briskly rub St 36 on the outside of your leg beneath your knee. Rub one side and then the other rapidly enough to make the skin feel warm and vibrant.

Step 7

Again hold Sp 16: Use your fingertips to support the base of your rib cage on both sides. Close your eyes and take long, slow, deep breaths into your abdomen for two minutes (see step 1).

Additional Points for Relieving Diarrhea

For illustrations of related points for relieving diarrhea, see chapter 6, "Anxiety and Nervousness"; chapter 32, "Motion Sickness, Morning Sickness, and Nausea"; and chapter 39, "Stomachaches, Indigestion, and Heartburn."

16
EARACHES

I will never forget the experience I had one time while on an airplane, showing Julie, a precious little nine year old, how to relieve her earaches. As we approached the San Francisco airport, and our altitude rapidly decreased, Julie covered her ears and began to cry. Her mother looked over at me anxiously and helplessly shook her head, "She always does this whenever we fly." Without even touching her, I showed Julie how to press the acupressure points underneath her earlobe to relieve the pain and pressure. She followed my instructions, and after a few minutes her pain was completely gone and she was smiling. Her mother was completely dazzled and grateful. This was the first time she had seen her daughter land without ear pain and with dry eyes!

Acupressure helps relieve earaches, as well as reduce inflammation. If you think your ear may be infected, however, acupressure is not the first treatment choice and you should always see a physician. If your ear is simply sensitive to cold or a change in air or water pressure, however, then acupressure can be effective.

The following acupressure points also relieve the pressure caused by water in the ear. They can be used effectively by children as well as adults.

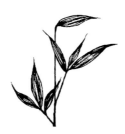

Potent Points for Relieving Earaches

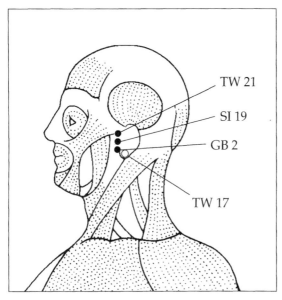

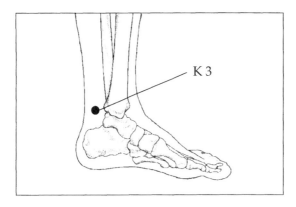

■ *You do not have to use all of these points. Using just one or two of them whenever you have a free hand can be effective.*

Ear Gate (TW 21)
Listening Place (SI 19)
Reunion of Hearing (GB 2)

Location: SI 19 is directly in front of the ear opening in a depression which will deepen when the mouth is open. TW 21 is one-half inch above this point and GB 2 is one-half inch below.

Benefits: Relieves earaches, hearing problems, pressure inside the ear, TMJ (jaw problems), toothaches, and headaches.

Wind Screen (TW 17)

Location: In the indentation behind the earlobe.

Benefits: Relieves ear pain, facial spasms, jaw pain, itchy ears, swollen throat, mumps, and toothaches.

Bigger Stream (K 3)
This last point is especially good for wisdom tooth pain.
Caution: This point is forbidden to be strongly stimulated after the third month of pregnancy.

Location: Midway between the inside of your anklebone and the Achilles tendon in the back of your ankle.

Benefits: Relieves earaches and ringing in the ears.

Potent Point Exercises

Lie down or sit in a comfortable position.

Step 1

Press TW 21, SI 19, and GB 2: Using your middle fingertips, find the middle point, SI 19, in the indentation that deepens when you open your mouth. Then place your ring finger directly above on TW 21 and your index finger directly on GB 2. Hold all three points together on both sides of your face for three minutes, with your mouth partially open and your eyes closed, while you concentrate on breathing deeply. If one of these points feels particularly connected to your earache, hold it for up to ten minutes or until the pain and pressure subside.

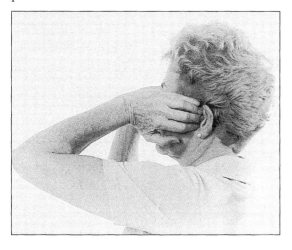

Step 2

Lightly press TW 17: Place your middle fingers in the hollows just behind the earlobes. Often these points are tender. Hold them lightly as you continue to breathe deeply for two minutes.

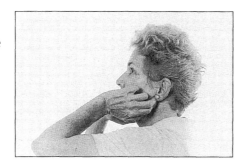

Step 3

Return to TW 21, SI 19, and GB 2: Again press these points in front of your ear and hold for a two more minutes as you take long, deep breaths.

Step 4

Press K 3: Finish the routine with a trigger point for relieving earaches. K 3 is located

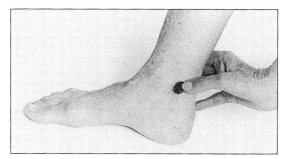

between the inside of your anklebone and the Achilles tendon, toward the back of your ankle. Use your right thumb to press the point on your right ankle and your left hand on your left ankle. Apply firm pressure for one minute on each side.

Repeat this routine three times daily. See your doctor if your earache does not go away after a couple of days.

17
EYESTRAIN

$\mathcal{A}$ number of factors can cause eyestrain, including overuse from driving, reading, watching television, or working at a computer monitor. Air pollution and fatigue can also cause or aggravate eyestrain. When your eyes feel achy or strained, it is often a signal that you're under stress and your whole body is tired. Other fatigue symptoms that usually accompany eyestrain include headaches, irritability, and tension in the back of the neck and shoulders.

Edward, a full-time computer programmer, began taking acupressure classes to help himself cope with on-the-job stress. He was quite withdrawn when it came to relating to other people. After learning the points for eyestrain, however, Edward's entire demeanor changed and he seemed more at ease.

The following self-help techniques and acupressure points for relieving eyestrain can help you feel better when you are weary, overworked, or tense.

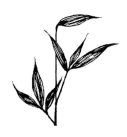

Potent Points for Relieving Eyestrain

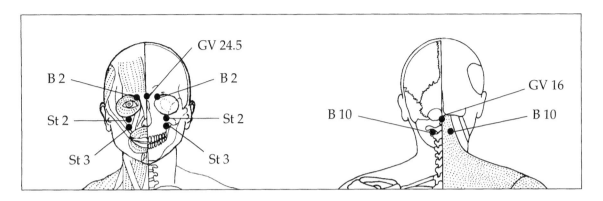

Drilling Bamboo (B 2)

Location: In the indentations outside of the bridge of the nose on the inner edge of the eyebrows.

Benefits: Relieves red and painful eyes, headaches, foggy vision, and hay fever.

Four Whites (St 2)

Location: One-half inch below the center of the lower eye ridge in an indentation of the cheek.

Benefits: Relieves burning or aching eyes, sinus pain, headaches, and dry eyes.

Facial Beauty (St 3)

Location: At the bottom of the cheekbone, directly in line with the pupil of the eye.

Benefits: Relieves eye fatigue and pressure, stuffy nose, and head congestion.

Heavenly Pillar (B 10)

Location: One-half inch below the base of the skull on the ropy muscles one-half inch outward from the spine.

Benefits: Relieves stress, burnout, exhaustion, heaviness in the head, eyestrain, and swollen eyes.

Wind Mansion (GV 16)

Location: At the top of the spinal column in the large hollow under the base of the skull.

Benefits: Aids the eyes, ears, nose, and throat; relieves mental problems and headaches.

Third Eye Point (GV 24.5)

Location: Directly between the eyebrows, in the indentation where the bridge of the nose meets the forehead.

Benefits: This helps the endocrine system, especially the pituitary gland, and relieves hay fever, headaches, and eyestrain.

Bigger Rushing (Lv 3)

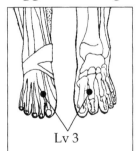

Location: On the top of the foot, in the webbing between the big toe and the second toe.

Benefits: Relieves headaches, tired eyes, and hangovers.

■ *You do not have to use all of these points. Using just one or two of them whenever you have a free hand can be effective.*

Potent Point Exercises

Wash your hands with soap and water to prevent eye infections before you begin this routine. Sit in a comfortable position as you hold each of the following acupressure points for at least one minute. Close your eyes and breathe deeply.

Step 1

Press B 2: Place your thumbs on the upper ridge of your eye sockets close to the bridge of your nose. Press upward into the indentations of the eye sockets as you breathe deeply for one minute.

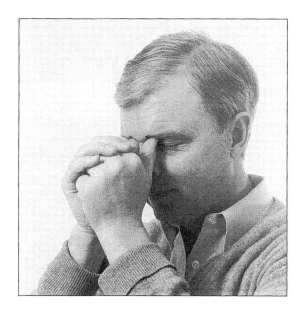

Step 2

Hold St 2 and St 3: Place your index fingers in the center of your cheeks below the lower ridge of your eyes, in line with the pupil. Then place your middle fingers directly below your index fingers, underneath the cheekbones. With your eyes closed, apply light pressure and breathe deeply for one minute.

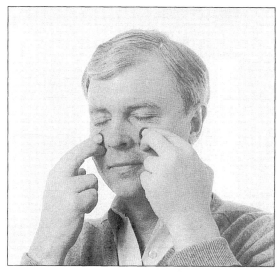

Step 3

Firmly press B 10: Curve your fingers to firmly press B 10 on the ropy muscles that run parallel to the spine. Hold for one minute as you breathe deeply.

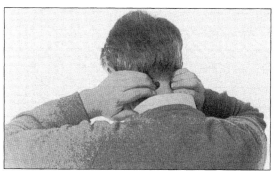

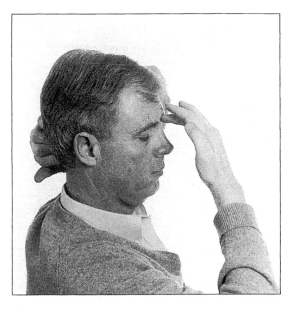

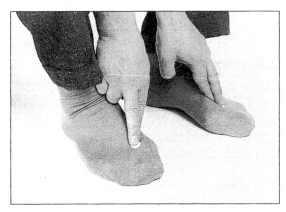

Step 4

Hold GV 16 and GV 24.5: Place the middle finger of your left hand on GV 16 in the large hollow in the middle of the base of your skull. Use the middle finger of your right hand to lightly touch GV 24.5 and focus your attention on that spot with your eyes closed. Breathe deeply as you hold this powerful healing point combination for one to two minutes.

Step 5

Stimulate Lv 3: Slip your shoes off. Starting between your large and second toes on both feet, slide your middle and index fingers up the top of the foot in the valley between the bones. Press firmly into the indentation just before the bones join to form a V shape. Rub back and forth against the skin to stimulate these eyestrain relief trigger points.

Additional Points for Relieving Eyestrain

For illustrations of other related points for relieving eyestrain, see chapter 16, "Earaches"; chapter 20, "Headaches and Migraines"; chapter 35, "Pain"; and chapter 38, "Sinus Problems and Hay Fever."

18
FAINTING

*T*he acupressure revival points for fainting stimulate the system to rebalance and rejuvenate the body. One of the most famous revival points is GV 26, located between the upper lip

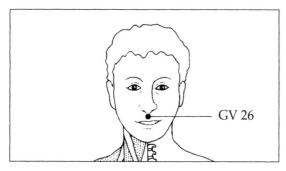

GV 26

and nose. You can use this point by itself or in conjunction with a series of other points to revive yourself instantly when you are feeling faint. The points also trigger the body's natural balancing mechanisms for restoring health.

I was at a friend's engagement party when another guest in his mid-teens, Frank, suddenly fainted. Apparently, he had been drinking champagne on an empty stomach. Fortunately, he fell against a couch and didn't break any bones. Before someone was able to reach a doctor, I pressed the acupressure point on the center of his upper gum directly below his nose and revived him. Frank's relatives were both grateful and impressed with the acupressure's effectiveness.

If you have a history of fainting due to general weakness, use the following points three times daily to strengthen your nervous system. If you experience recurring fainting or convulsions, however, always consult a physician.

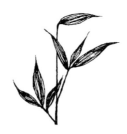

Potent Points for Relieving Fainting

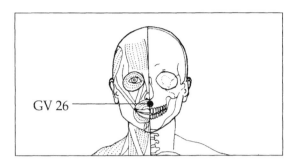

Middle of a Person (GV 26)

Location: Two-thirds of the way up from the upper lip to the nose.

Benefits: This first-aid revival point has traditionally been used for relieving cramps, fainting, dizziness, epilepsy, spinal pain, and extreme emotional agitation.

Sea of Vitality (B 23 and B 47)

Caution: Do not press on disintegrating discs or fractured or broken bones. If you have a weak back, a few minutes of stationary, light touching instead of pressure can be very healing. See your doctor first if you have any questions or need medical advice.

Location: On either side of the lower back two and four finger widths away from the spine at waist level.

Benefits: Relieves fainting, dizziness, fatigue, extreme weakness, and instability.

Bubbling Springs (K 1)

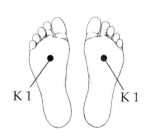

Location: On the sole of the foot in the center between the two pads.

Benefits: First-aid point for relieving fainting, shock, and convulsions.

Three Mile Point (St 36)

Location: Four finger widths below the kneecap, one finger width outside of the shinbone. If you are on the correct spot, a muscle should flex as you move your foot up and down.

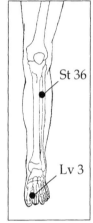

Benefits: Strengthens the whole body, tones the muscles, and grounds a person when weak, tired, dizzy, or faint.

Bigger Rushing (Lv 3)

Location: On the top of the foot, in the valley between the big toe and second toe.

Benefits: Relieves fainting, dizziness, exhaustion, headaches, minor nervous disorders, and hangovers.

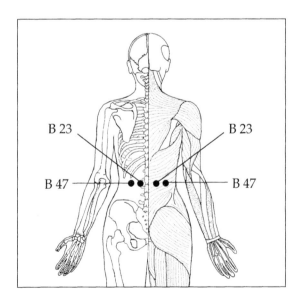

■ *You do not have to use all of these points. Using just one or two of them whenever you have a free hand can be effective.*

Potent Point Exercises

Sit in a comfortable position.

Step 1

Firmly press GV 26: Use your index finger to press between the base of your nose and your upper lip. Press deeply, applying firm pressure to the center of your upper gum for one minute.

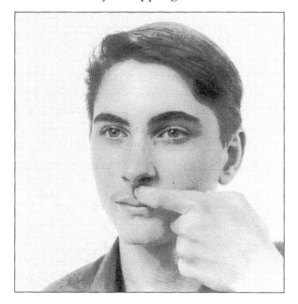

Step 2

Rub B 23 and B 47: Make fists and place your knuckles against your lower back. Rapidly rub up and down for one minute to stimulate these vitality points.

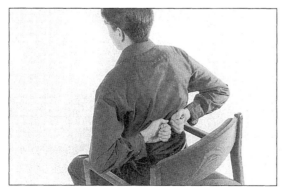

Slip off your shoes to complete this routine.

Step 3

Briskly rub St 36: Place your right heel on St 36 of your left leg and briskly rub it for one minute. Then do the same on your other leg. This will both revive and strengthen your whole system.

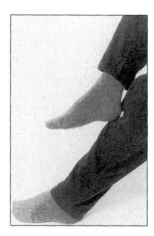

Step 4

Rub Lv 3: Place both of your middle and index fingers in between your large and second toes on top of your feet. Briskly rub for thirty seconds in the groove between the two bones that join these toes.

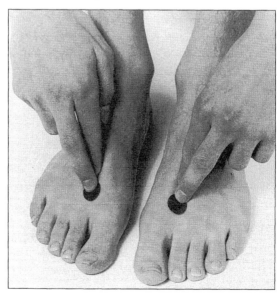

Step 5

Press or rub K 1:
Make a fist and rub the sole of your foot for thirty seconds. Then use your other hand to rub the bottom of your opposite foot. Or, if you prefer, simply hold K 1 with your thumb or fingertips. Pressing this first-aid point gives you a quick way to pick yourself up when you're feeling fatigued or faint.

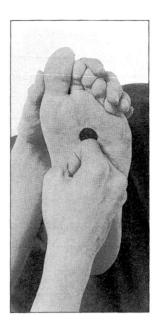

Additional Points for Relieving Fainting

For illustrations of other related points for relieving fainting, see chapter 10, "Chronic Fatigue Syndrome"; chapter 23, "Immune System Boosting"; and chapter 30, "Memory and Concentration."

19

HANGOVERS

*A*cupressure can relieve many of the discomforts of a hangover: throbbing headache, eye pain, hypersensitivity, nausea, and fatigue. It increases blood circulation and releases muscular tension. Naturally, when the blood and energy circulate properly, the entire system functions better and we have a greater sense of health and well-being. The increased circulation also enables the body to detoxify itself and relieves hangovers.

Although this chapter illustrates the key points to relieve hangovers, these same points can be used for those who need to balance their systems and readjust their behaviors so that they can overcome alcoholic tendencies.

If you have had a history of drinking or are tempted to drink, but don't want to, practicing self-acupressure twice a day for three weeks may reduce your craving. Of course, it is wise to seek professional counseling and assistance from a support group such as Alcoholics Anonymous to help you change other attitudes and behaviors.

A friend of mine, whom I met playing football, was helped immensely by the following potent point recovery routine. When pressed once or twice a day, the acupressure points help to release muscular contractions and pressures associated with hangovers to restore balance to the body.

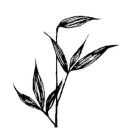

Potent Points for Relieving Hangovers

Joining the Valley (Hoku) (LI 4)

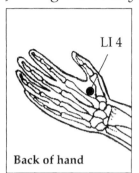

LI 4

Back of hand

Caution: This point is forbidden for pregnant women until labor because its stimulation can cause premature contractions in the uterus.

Location: In the webbing between the thumb and index finger, at the highest spot of the muscle that protrudes when the thumb and index finger are brought close together.

Benefits: Relieves pain (in general), especially frontal headaches due to hangovers, shoulder pain, and labor pain.

Heavenly Pillar (B 10)

Location: One-half inch below the base of the skull, on the ropy muscles one-half inch outward from the spine.

Benefits: Relieves stress, burnout, exhaustion, insomnia, heaviness in the head, eyestrain, stiff necks, and sore throats.

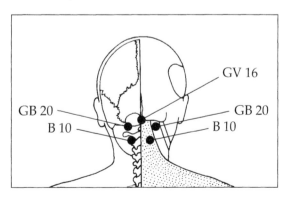

■ *You do not have to use all of these points. Using just one or two of them whenever you have a free hand can be effective.*

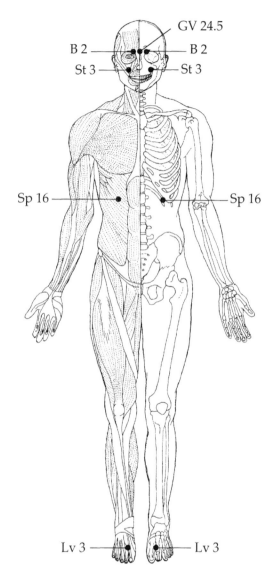

Gates of Consciousness (GB 20)

Location: Below the base of the skull, in the hollows between the two major neck muscles, two to three inches apart depending on the size of the head.

Benefits: Relieves eye pain, throbbing headaches, dizziness, stiff neck, coordination problems, and irritability.

98

Abdominal Sorrow (Sp 16)
Location: On the lower edge of the rib cage one-half inch in from the nipple line.

Benefits: Relieves hangovers, nausea, ulcer pain, indigestion, appetite imbalances, abdominal cramps, and hiccups.

Bigger Rushing (Lv 3)
Location: On the top of the foot, in the valley between the big toe and the second toe.

Benefits: Relieves headaches, tired eyes, hangovers, allergies, and arthritis.

Third Eye Point (GV 24.5)
Location: Directly between the eyebrows, in the indentation where the bridge of the nose meets the forehead.

Benefits: Relieves headaches, indigestion, and low morale; helps those who feel their spiritual growth is blocked.

Wind Mansion (GV 16)
Location: In the center of the back of the head in the large hollow under the base of the skull.

Benefits: Relieves hangovers, headaches, vertigo, stiff necks, head congestion, and mental stress.

Facial Beauty (St 3)
Location: At the bottom of the cheekbone, directly below the pupil.

Benefits: Relieves head congestion, burning eyes, and bloodshot or swollen eyes.

Drilling Bamboo (B 2)
Location: In the indentations on either side of where the bridge of the nose meets the ridge of the eyebrows.

Benefits: Relieves hangovers, red and painful eyes, headaches, foggy vision, sinus pain, hay fever, and head congestion.

Potent Point Exercises

Sit comfortably.

Step 1
Grasp LI 4: Spread your thumb and index finger apart as you press into the muscle of the web, and angle the pressure slightly toward the bone that connects with the index finger. Stimulate each side for one minute.

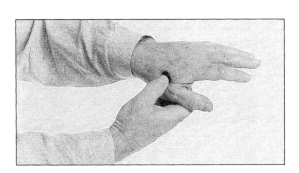

Step 2
Firmly press B 10:
Curve your fingers to press the thick, ropy muscles on the back of your upper neck. Breathe deeply as you hold for one minute.

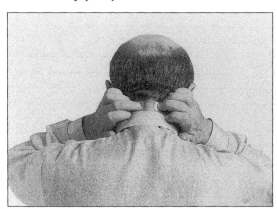

Step 3

Press GB 20: Place your thumbs underneath the base of your skull, in the hollow spots about two inches apart. Close your eyes and gradually tilt your head back as you apply firm pressure underneath the skull for at least one minute or until you feel a regular, even pulse on both sides. Then hold lightly to encourage the point to open and pulsate.

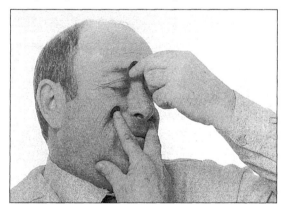

Step 4

Hold both points B 2 with St 3: Place the thumb and index finger of one hand on the upper ridge of the eye socket (B 2) near the bridge of your nose. Press up into the

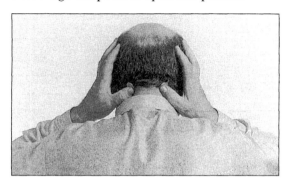

indentations in your eye socket. Then spread the index and middle finger of your other hand to press St 3 up underneath your cheekbones directly beneath your eyes. Hold this point combination for one minute with your eyes closed as you breathe deeply.

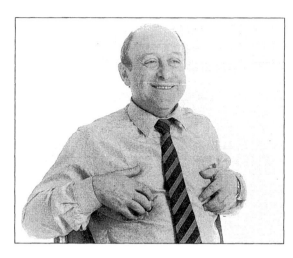

Step 5

Hold Sp 16: Curve your fingers to press on the base of your ribcage on the line beneath the nipple. Gently press upward into the slight indentations on the bottom edge of the rib cage for one minute as you take long deep breaths through your nose.

Step 6

Hold GV 16 with GV 24.5: Place your right thumb in the center of the skull pressing into a large hollow (GV 16). Use the third finger of your left hand to touch GV 24.5, in the indentation between your eyebrows. Hold these points for a minute with your eyes closed, focusing your attention at the Third Eye Point. Breath deeply to clear your mind.

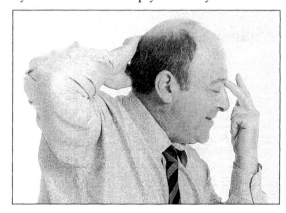

Step 7

Upper back opener exercise: Stand up and interlace your fingers behind the base of your spine. Slowly bring your upper body forward and down as your arms stretch upward. Take a couple of deep breaths in this position, then relax your arms, letting them swing back and forth several times. Bend your knees and slowly come back to a relaxed standing position. This stretching exercise brings blood to the head and increases the circulation.

Slip off your shoes off and sit down comfortably to work on the last point.

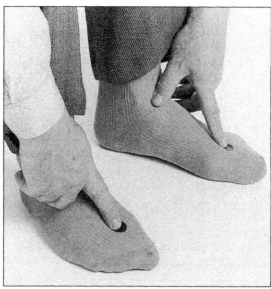

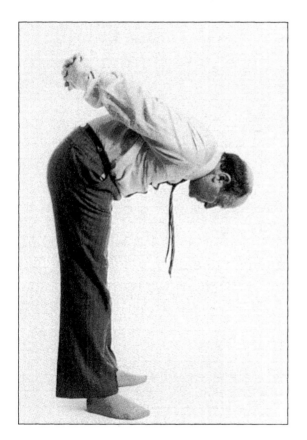

Step 8

Stimulate Lv 3: Reach down to place your index fingers between your big toe and second toe. Slide your finger two inches toward your leg in an indentation between the bones on the top of your feet: Press firmly on an angle toward the bone that attaches to the second toe or simply rub briskly for thirty seconds. This is an excellent decongestant point for clearing the head.

Additional Points for Relieving Hangovers

For illustrations of other related points for relieving hangovers, see chapter 17, "Eyestrain"; chapter 20, "Headaches and Migraines"; chapter 26, "Irritability, Frustration and Dealing with Change"; and chapter 37, "Shoulder Tension."

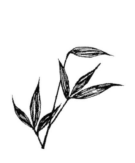

20
HEADACHES AND MIGRAINES

$\mathcal{M}$ost headaches are caused primarily by tension in the muscles of the head, neck, and shoulders, which constricts the blood vessels that supply oxygen to the nerve cells in the brain. A headache is the body's warning signal that the brain may not be getting enough oxygen. Too often, we choose to repress these signals by taking aspirin, instead of relieving the stress or muscle tension causing the headache. If you have a bad headache that persists for more than several days, you should always call your doctor.

Migraine headaches involve intense pain and often are accompanied by nausea and visual disorders. It is a serious condition for which you should be under a physician's care. But acupressure can be an effective complementary treatment to treat the pain of migraines. Larry, one my clients, is a general contractor who occasionally suffers from migraine headaches. He asked me once what he could do to relieve them himself although he was continuing to take his medication. I showed him two potent points: one in the pit of the stomach, two inches directly above the navel, the other on the top of the foot in the groove between the bones of the fourth and fifth toes. A few weeks later, Larry told me that he had used these points for a throbbing, full-blown migraine headache while at a builder's conference — and that most of his symptoms had receded in just five minutes!

I recently had a date with my friend Carrie, who developed a splitting headache shortly after a call from her parents upset her. I worked on her shoulders and neck, then underneath the base of her skull, the bridge of her nose, and finally her feet. At one point she took a deep breath and let out a sigh and said she realized how she needed to deal with her parents. After the half-hour acupressure session, Carrie told me her headache was gone and that she felt like her old self again.

From a Chinese health care perspective, headaches and other symptoms are not only considered expressions of a physical condition, but also the emotional and spiritual aspects of the person as a whole. Acupressure can help uncover the reasons behind recurring headaches.

Common Causes of Headaches

Misalignment: If the vertebrae of the neck are out of alignment, they throw off the position of the head, creating strain on neck and head muscles. Misaligned vertebrae can cause discs to "pinch" a neck nerve and cause headaches. If you have severe pain, you should always see a physician.

Minor cervical misalignments and headaches can be relieved by pressing B 10, on the ropy muscles on the upper neck one-half inch out from the spine. Lie on your back and hold B 10, firmly supporting your neck muscles, for three minutes as you breathe deeply. Then bring your hands by your sides, close your eyes, and let yourself completely relax for five minutes.

Intestinal Congestion: Frontal headaches are often accompanied by constipation. The point LI 4, Joining the Valley (Hoku),[32] located

---

[32] Caution: Forbidden for pregnant women until labor because its stimulation can cause premature contractions in the uterus. To relieve headaches during pregnancy, close your eyes and massage the points in the temples, bridge of the nose, and the base of the skull (see pages 90-92). Then apply firm but gentle pressure to the bottoms and tops of your feet between the bones of your toes. End the routine by stimulating your toes.

in the webbing between the thumb and index finger, helps relieve congestion in both the head and the digestive system. Pressing this point on each hand for two minutes relieves frontal headaches.

Abdominal massage also relieves both constipation and headaches. Press points in a circle three inches from the navel (picture a clock, and press one point for each number on the clock). Work in a clockwise direction (facing the abdomen).

Sinus Headaches: When fluids in the back of your nose are unable to drain, pressure builds up in the sinus cavities and causes headaches. Use point B 2, then St 3, and finally, Lv 3, to relieve sinus blockage and headache. All three points are described on the pages that follow.

Potent Points for Relieving Headaches and Migraines

Gates of Consciousness (GB 20)

Location: Below the base of the skull, in the hollow between the two vertical neck muscles.

Benefits: Relieves arthritis, headaches (including migraines), dizziness, stiff neck, neck pain, neuromotor coordination problems, eyestrain, and irritability.

Wind Mansion (GV 16)

Location: In the center of the back of the head in a large hollow under the base of the skull.

Benefits: Relieves pain in the eyes, ears, nose, and throat, as well as mental problems, headaches, vertigo, and stiff necks.

Drilling Bamboo (B 2)

Location: In the indentations on either side of where the bridge of the nose meets the ridge of the eyebrows.

Benefits: Relieves eye pain, headaches, hay fever, eye fatigue, and sinus pain.

Third Eye Point (GV 24.5)

Location: Directly between the eyebrows, in the indentation where the bridge of the nose meets the forehead.

Benefits: This point balances the pituitary gland, and relieves hay fever, headaches, indigestion, ulcer pain, and eyestrain.

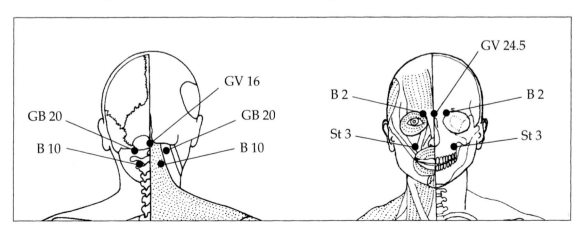

Facial Beauty (St 3)

Location: At the bottom of the cheekbone, below the pupil.

Benefits: Relieves eye fatigue and pressure, nasal and head congestion, eyestrain, and toothaches.

Joining the Valley (Hoku) (LI 4)

Caution: This point is forbidden for pregnant women because its stimulation can cause premature contractions in the uterus.

Location: In the webbing between the thumb and index finger, at the highest spot of the muscle that protrudes when the thumb and index finger are brought close together.

Benefits: Relieves frontal headaches, toothaches, shoulder pain, and labor pain.

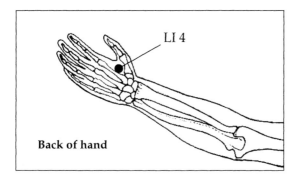

Bigger Rushing (Lv 3)

Location: On the top of the foot, in the valley between the big toe and second toe.

Benefits: Relieves foot cramps, headaches, eye fatigue, hangovers, allergies, and arthritis.

Above Tears (GB 41)

Location: On the top of the foot, one inch above the webbing of the fourth and fifth toes in the groove between the bones.

Benefits: Relieves hip pain, shoulder tension, arthritic pains that move all over the body, headaches, sideaches, water retention, and sciatica.

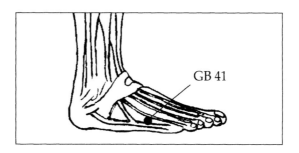

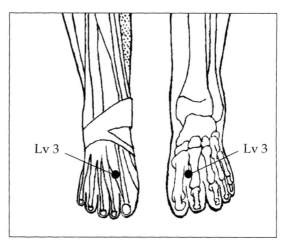

■ *You do not have to use all of these points. Using just one or two of them whenever you have a free hand can be effective.*

Potent Point Exercises

*The following routine can be done
either lying down or sitting comfortably.*

Step 1

Rub your head, then press your stomach:
Use your fingertips to briskly rub all parts of
your skull, as if you were shampooing your
hair, for one minute. Then place your
fingertips two inches directly above your belly
button and gradually press into the pit of your
stomach while you breathe deeply for one
minute.

Step 2

Firmly press GB 20: Use your thumbs to
press underneath the base of your skull into
the hollow areas on either side, two to three
inches apart depending on the size of your
head. Slowly tilt your head back with your
eyes closed, and firmly press up underneath
the skull for one to two minutes as you take
long, deep breaths. This is something you can
teach your child.

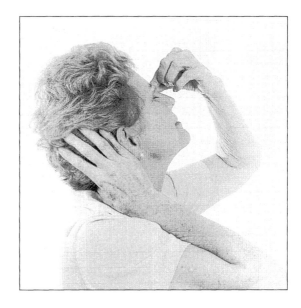

Step 3

Hold GV 16 with B 2: Use your right thumb
to press GV 16 in the center hollow at the base
of the skull. Use your left thumb and index
finger to press B 2 in the upper hollows of the
eye socket near the bridge of the nose. Again,
tilt your head back and breathe deeply for one
or two minutes.

Step 4

Lightly press GV 24.5: With the palms
of your hands together, let your head tilt

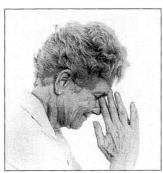

downward and
position your
index and third
fingers on
GV 24.5. Con-
centrate on this
spot for two
minutes as you
breathe deeply.

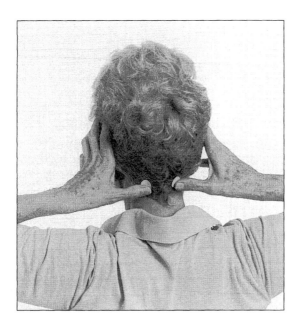

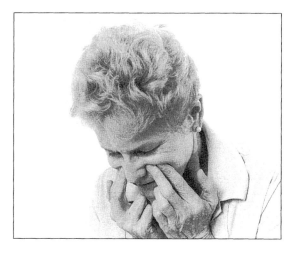

Step 5

Press St 3: Use your middle and index fingers on both hands to gently press up underneath the cheekbones, directly below the center of your eyes, for one minute.

Step 6

Firmly press LI 4: Place your right hand over the top of your left hand. Use your right thumb to press the webbing between the thumb and index finger of your left hand. Angle the pressure toward the bone that connects with the index finger. Hold for one minute. Then press this point for one minute on your opposite hand.

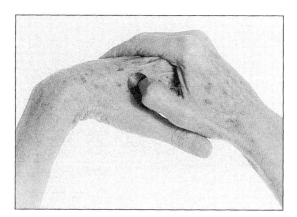

Slip off your shoes and sit down comfortably to work on these last two trigger points for relieving headaches.

Step 7

Stimulate Lv 3 and GB 41: Place your right heel on top of your left foot to rub in between the bones on the tops of your feet for one minute. Stimulate the sensitive spots between your big and second toe as well as between the bones that connect to your fourth and little toes. Then switch and work on the opposite foot.

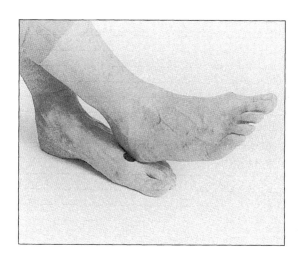

Additional Points for Relieving Headaches and Migraines

For illustrations of other related points for relieving headaches and migraines, see chapter 17, "Eyestrain"; chapter 19, "Hang-overs"; chapter 33, "Neck Tension, Whiplash and Pain"; and chapter 35, "Pain."

21
HICCUPS

I will never forget the time when my mother was unable to get rid of her hiccups. She had been in the kitchen with my sister trying numerous approaches, but after ten or fifteen minutes, she was at her wit's end. I asked her if I could hold a few spots at the base of her ribs, and after a couple of minutes, her hiccups stopped. I have been able to help a number of other people — at parties as well as conventions — relieve this annoying condition.

Hiccups are rhythmic spasms in the diaphragm, lungs, and sometimes the throat. Usually just a few minutes of finger pressure triggers a relaxation response in the throat, lungs, and diaphragm. The combination of abdominal breathing with acupressure and relaxation is key to relieving hiccups. Therefore, it's important to make yourself comfortable and breathe deeply while holding the following acupressure points.

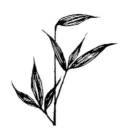

Potent Points for Relieving Hiccups

Wind Screen (TW 17)

Location: In the indentation behind the ear lobe.

Benefits: Relieves hiccups as well as ear pain, facial paralysis, facial spasms, jaw pain, damp and itchy ears, swollen throats, mumps, and toothaches. Holding this point on both sides and taking slow, deep breaths is one of the fastest ways to relieve hiccups.

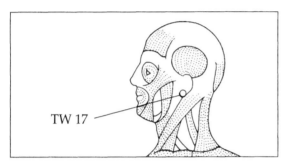

TW 17

Abdominal Sorrow (Sp 16)

Location: On the lower edge of the rib cage (at the junction of the ninth rib cartilage to the eighth rib), one-half inch in from the nipple line.

Benefits: Relieves hiccups, indigestion, appetite imbalances, abdominal cramps, and ulcer pain.

Heaven Rushing Out (CV 22)

Location: At the base of the throat in the center of the collarbones.

Benefits: Relieves hiccups, bronchitis, throat spasms, sore throats, chest congestion, and heartburn.

Sea of Tranquility (CV 17)

Location: On the center of the breastbone three thumb widths up from the base of the bone.

Benefits: Relieves nervousness, anxiety, panic attacks, and hiccups.

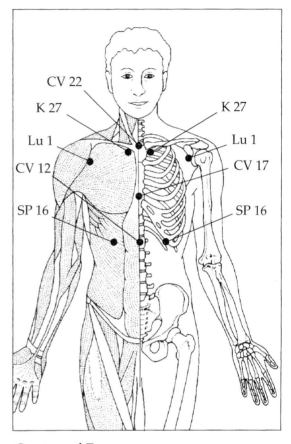

CV 22
K 27
Lu 1
CV 12
SP 16

K 27
Lu 1
CV 17
SP 16

Center of Power (CV 12)

Caution: Do not hold this point deeply if you have a serious illness. See caution on page 9. Even if you are not ill, however, it is best not to hold this point for more than two minutes and to use it only on a fairly empty stomach.

Location: On the midline of the body, three finger widths below the base of the breastbone, in the pit of the upper stomach.

Benefits: Relieves hiccups, abdominal spasms, indigestion, heartburn, constipation, emotional stress, and headaches.

■ *You do not have to use all of these points. Using just one or two of them whenever you have a free hand can be effective.*

Letting Go (Lu 1)

Location: On the outer part of the chest, two inches above the crease of the armpit and one inch inward. When you pull your arm close to your body you should feel a muscle bulge.

Benefits: Relieves hiccups, breathing difficulties, and coughing.

Elegant Mansion (K 27)

Location: In the hollow below the collarbone next to the breastbone.

Benefits: Relieves chest congestion, breathing difficulties, asthma, coughing, hiccups, and anxiety.

Potent Point Exercises

The following routine helps both prevent and relieve your hiccups. Usually applying just the first three steps, which take three or four minutes, will stop the hiccups. Lie down or sit comfortably and breathe deeply as you hold each of the following points.

Step 1

Lightly press TW 17: Place your middle and index fingers behind each earlobe. This point is usually ultrasensitive to finger pressure. Lightly hold these tender points for one minute.

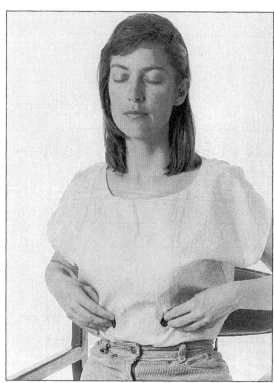

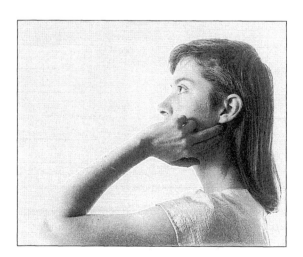

Step 2

Firmly hold Sp 16: Curve your fingers to hold the base of your rib cage directly below your nipples. Close your eyes and breathe deeply for one minute as you gently press up into the indentations at the base of your ribs.

Step 3

Hold CV 22 and CV 17: Place your right middle finger in the hollow at the base of your throat, gently directing pressure downward. Use all the fingers of your left hand to firmly hold the center of your breastbone in the slight indentations of the breastbone. Close your eyes and take long, deep breaths for one full minute.

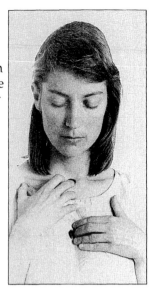

Step 5

Firmly press K 27: Place your fingertips in the indentations directly below the protrusions of your collarbone. Press firmly for thirty seconds as you take a long, deep breath.

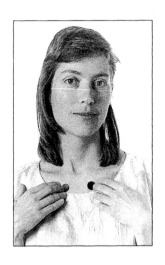

Step 6

Press Lu 1 firmly: Use your thumbs to apply pressure to the upper, outer portion of your chest, feeling for a "knot" of tension. Again breathe deeply as you hold this point for one minute.

Step 4

Gradually press CV 12: Place all of your fingers in the center of your abdomen between your belly button and the base of your breastbone. Slowly apply the pressure at an upward angle toward the center of your back. Breathe deeply as you hold for one minute.

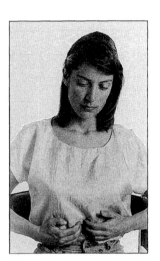

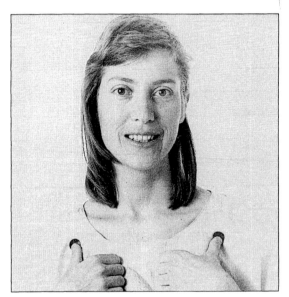

Additional Points for Relieving Hiccups

For illustrations of other related points for relieving hiccups, see chapter 6, "Anxiety and Nervousness"; and chapter 8, "Asthma and Breathing Difficulties."

22
HOT FLASHES

Carol, a proud mother of three and a former executive secretary, complained of hot flashes when she began her training at the Acupressure Institute. Carol inspired me to write this chapter because she relieved her hot flashes simply by taking classes and practicing the points on herself for two months. This chapter highlights the most important points Carol used on herself.

Hot flashes and cold feet are some of the common symptoms of menopause. Hot flashes can also result from arteriosclerosis and imbalances in the autonomic system. They commonly occur under stressful circumstances — when a person is giving a presentation before a large group of people, for instance. Most people who suffer from hot flashes also develop high blood pressure and experience anxiety, insomnia, headaches, and irritability.

Hot flashes due to menopause occur when estrogen levels in the ovaries suddenly decrease. Estrogen is regulated by the pituitary gland in the brain. The area of the brain that regulates body temperature — sort of the body's "thermostat" — lies near the area that controls both ovary and pituitary hormone production. Research related to hot flashes has shown that the neurotransmitter known as norepinephrine that stimulates these brain mechanisms also affects this thermostat in the brain.

Although hot flashes are usually most intense during the first two years after menopause begins, some women have experienced the heat discomfort for up to nine years. When a woman has hot flashes at night, they can disturb her sleep, causing fatigue and irritability the next day.

Women commonly find that hot drinks and meals, alcohol, coffee, hot weather, and a warm room trigger hot flashes. Emotional stress and caffeine both are significant contributing factors. Caffeine especially has been found to raise the metabolism and increase body temperature. It also triggers the release of norepinephrine. As preventive measures, keep yourself relatively cool, don't overdress, and avoid both alcohol and caffeine.

Stress reduction practices such as acupressure, gentle stretching, and breathing exercises lower norepinephrine levels, reducing or even preventing hot flashes.[33] Using the following acupressure points one to four times each day balances the body, stabilizes blood pressure, and reduces flushing.

---

[33] Sadja Greenwood, M.D., *Menopause Naturally* (Volcano: Volcano Press, 1989), 30.

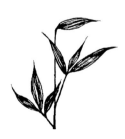

Potent Points for Relieving Hot Flashes

Bubbling Springs (K 1)

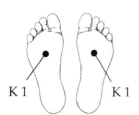

Location: At the base of the ball of the foot, between the two pads.

Benefits: Relieves hot flashes, fainting, and convulsions.

Elegant Mansion (K 27)

Location: In the hollow below the collarbone next to the breastbone.

Benefits: Relieves hot flashes as well as chest congestion, breathing difficulties, asthma, coughing, anxiety, and depression.

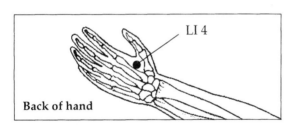

Back of hand

Joining the Valley (Hoku) (LI 4)

Caution: This point is forbidden for pregnant women because its stimulation can cause premature contractions in the uterus.

Location: In the webbing between the thumb and index finger at the highest spot of the muscle when the thumb and index finger are brought close together.

Benefits: Relieves hot flashes and is a trigger point for arthritis in the hand, headaches, and toothaches.

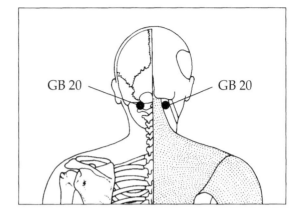

Gates of Consciousness (GB 20)

Location: Below the base of the skull, in the hollows two or three inches apart depending on the size of the head.

Benefits: Relieves hot flashes as well as headaches, dizziness, stiff neck, neck pain, injuries, trauma, shock, hypertension, and irritability.

Sea of Tranquility (CV 17)

Location: On the center of the breastbone three thumb widths up from the base of the bone.

Benefits: Relieves hot flashes as well as nervousness, anxiety, insomnia, depression, and emotional distress.

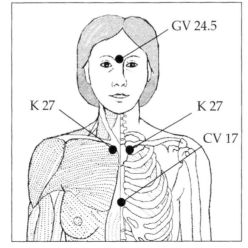

■ *You do not have to use all of these points. Using just one or two of them whenever you have a free hand can be effective.*

Third Eye Point
(GV 24.5)

Location: Directly between the eyebrows, in the indentation where the bridge of the nose meets the forehead.

Benefits: This acupressure point helps the endocrine system, especially the pituitary gland, and relieves hot flashes, hay fever, and headaches.

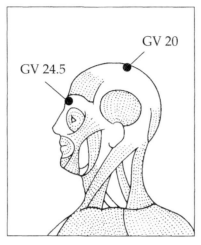

One Hundred Meeting Point (GV 20)

Location: On the crown of the head in an indentation or "soft spot" between the cranial bones. To find the point, follow the line from the back of the ears to the top of the head.

Benefits: This point improves mental concentration and memory; relieves headaches, hot flashes, and heatstroke.

Potent Point Exercises

Lie down or sit comfortably and breathe deeply as you hold each of the following points.

Step 1

Press K 1: Use your thumb to gradually press K 1 on the bottom of your left foot. Hold for a minute and then switch sides to press K 1 on your right foot.

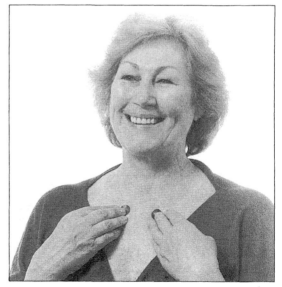

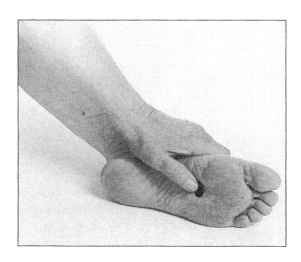

Step 2

Firmly hold both K 27 points: Place your third fingers in the indentations directly below the protrusions of your collarbone on your chest. Press firmly as you take slow, deep breaths for one minute.

115

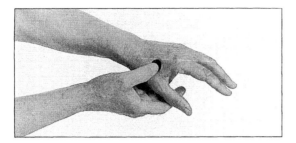

Step 3

Grasp LI 4: Place your right thumb on the webbing on the top of your left hand, with your fingertips on the underside directly below your thumb. Squeeze the thumb and index finger of your right hand together to firmly press into the webbing. Angle the pressure toward the bone that connects with your left index finger. Hold for one minute, and then switch sides.

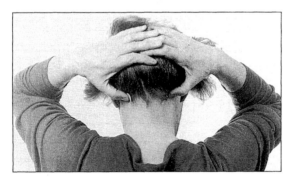

Step 4

Firmly press GB 20: Place your thumbs underneath the base of your skull into the hollow spots two to three inches apart depending on the size of your head. Slowly tilt your head back and breathe deeply. Apply pressure gradually, holding firmly for one minute as you focus on taking long, slow, deep breaths.

Step 5

Touch GV 20 and GV 24.5: Use the fingertips of your right hand to press GV 20 in the slight hollow at the rear of the top of your head.

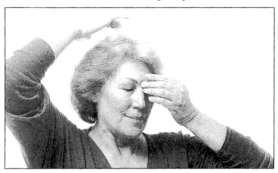

Place the middle fingertip of your left hand lightly in between your eyebrows on GV 24.5 in an indentation called the Third Eye Point. Focus your attention on that spot with your eyes closed. Straighten your spine and breathe deeply for two minutes as you hold these nervous system balancing points.

Step 6

Hold CV 17: Place all your fingertips on the center of your breastbone at heart level, fitting them into each of the indentations. Close your eyes, and breathe deeply for one minute.

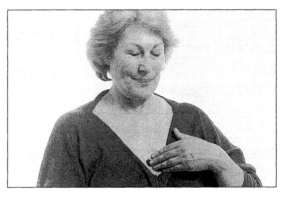

Additional Points for Relieving Hot Flashes

For illustrations of other related points for relieving hot flashes, see chapter 6, "Anxiety and Nervousness"; chapter 14, "Depression and Emotional Balancing"; chapter 20, "Headaches and Migraines"; and chapter 26, "Irritability, Frustration and Dealing with Change."

23
Immune System Boosting

*I*n a fast-paced world, it is easy to overwork yourself, take on too many commitments, and extend yourself to the point of exhaustion. This energy imbalance weakens the immune system. If we take care of ourselves by eating properly, getting enough rest and exercise, and practicing techniques that release tension and balance our bodies — then our resistance to illness is strong. If, on the other hand, we abuse our bodies, push ourselves too hard, eat poorly, don't exercise, and fail to release tension, our immune system weakens, and we are more prone to illness. Acupressure and deep breathing strengthen the immune system and can you help ward off disease.

Everyday stresses accumulate inside our bodies, causing shoulder and neck tensions as well as anxieties that often make it hard to breathe. I use acupressure, deep breathing, and stretching exercises daily to counteract the common daily pressures in my life.

We can only withstand a certain amount of stress. Each person has a different threshold and each must determine for himself or herself how much is too much. When you cultivate an inner awareness of what's going on inside you, both emotionally and physically, you discover your optimum balance of activity and rest.

Traditional Chinese medicine discovered that excesses of particular activities weaken the immune system by overstressing certain acupressure meridian pathways. (The following potent points are described in detail later in this chapter.)

- **Excess *standing*** damages the bladder and kidney meridians, which can cause fatigue and low backaches. To restore these meridians, stimulate the Sea of Vitality points (B 23

and B 47) by rubbing your lower back for one minute. Then hold Elegant Mansion (K 27) directly below your collarbone for another minute. Finally, hold the Bigger Stream (K 3) points on the insides of your ankles for one minute as you breathe deeply.

- **Excess *sitting*** can damage the stomach and spleen meridians, which can contribute to anemia or digestive disorders. Stimulate the Three Mile Points (St 36) on the outsides of your calves to benefit these meridians.

- **Excess *lying down*** can damage the large intestine and lung meridians, which can affect both respiration and elimination. For these meridians use Joining the Valley (Hoku, LI 4) in the valley between the thumb and forefinger and Crooked Pond (LI 11) on the upper edge of your elbow crease as directed on page 120.

- **Excess *use of your eyes*** (as in close desk work) or ***emotional stress*** can damage the small intestine and heart meridians, which can create emotional imbalances. The Sea of Tranquility (CV 17) on the center of your breastbone is an excellent point for balancing these meridians.

- **Excess *physical exertion*** can damage the gallbladder and liver meridians, which can cause cramps and spasms. Use Bigger Rushing (Lv 3) on the top of your feet to benefit these meridians.

By using these acupressure points regularly, balancing your activities, and practicing deep breathing you can counteract stresses, prevent fatigue, and boost your immune system. Deep breathing exercises alone can greatly increase your energy level and boost your immune system (see page 123).

Diet also plays an important role in building resistance to illness. When we eat processed, preserved, or devitalized foods, we weaken our immune system and our resistance because these foods have been stripped of necessary nutrients and fiber. Certain foods, such as miso soup, parsley, beans, tofu, sea vegetables, fresh vegetables, and lightly toasted sesame seeds, can strengthen the immune system and reinforce the body's ability to protect itself.

Acupressure Points for Strengthening the Immune System

There is a particular acupressure point, Bearing Support (B 36), that governs resistance, especially resistance to colds and flu. It

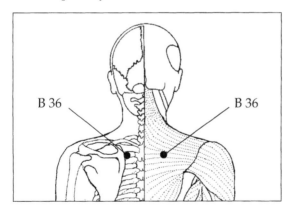

is located near the spine, off the tips of the shoulder blades. The Chinese book *The Yellow Emperor's Classic of Internal Medicine* says, "wind and cold enter the pores of the skin" at this point.[34] It, as well as other points in this area, helps to strengthen the immune system.

Conversely, these points around the tips of the shoulder blades are the first to get blocked up just before an illness, especially a cold or flu, takes hold.

The following acupressure points are effective for dealing with a condition that may be caused by a weak immune system. Elegant Mansion (K 27) reinforces immune system functioning by strengthening the respiratory system. Steady, firm pressure on the Sea of Vitality points (B 23 and B 47) fortifies the immune system, rejuvenates the internal organs, and relieves pain associated with lower back problems. The Sea of Energy (CV 6) tones the abdominal muscles and intestines, and helps fortify the immune, urinary, and reproductive systems. Firm pressure on the Three Mile Point (St 36) immediately boosts the immune system with renewed energy. It helps tone and strengthen the major muscle groups, providing greater endurance. Bigger Stream (K 3) on the inside of the ankle helps balance the kidney meridian and strengthen the immune system. Bigger Rushing (Lv 3) and Crooked Pond (LI 11) are important points for relieving pain and strengthening the immune system. The Outer Gate point (TW 5) helps to balance the immune system and strengthen the whole body. Hoku (LI 4) is a famous decongestant and anti-inflammatory point; it relieves arthritic pain and strengthens the immune system. Last, and most important of all, the Sea of Tranquility (CV 17) governs the body's resistance to illness and decreases anxiety by regulating the thymus gland. Each of these important points benefits the immune system by enabling the internal organs to function at optimal levels.

---

[34] Felix Mann, *Treatment of Disease by Acupuncture* (London: Heinemann Medical Books, 1967), 32, 37.

Potent Points for Boosting the Immune System

Elegant Mansion (K 27)

Location: In the depression directly below the protrusions of the collarbone.

Benefits: Strengthens the immune system as well as relieves chest congestion, breathing difficulties, asthma, coughing, anxiety, and depression.

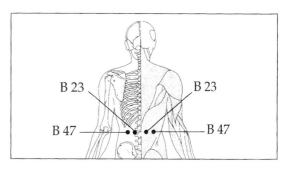

Sea of Vitality (B 23 and B 47)

Caution: Do not press on disintegrating discs or fractured or broken bones. If you have a weak back, a few minutes of stationary, light touching instead of pressure can be very healing. See your doctor first if you have any questions or need medical advice.

Location: In the lower back, between the second and third lumbar vertebrae, two to four finger widths away from the spine at waist level.

Benefits: Fortifies the immune system as well as relieves lower-back aches and fatigue.

Sea of Energy (CV 6)

Location: Two finger widths below the belly button, between it and the pubic bone.

Benefits: Strengthens the condition of the immune system and the internal organs as well as relieves abdominal muscle pain, constipation, gas, and general weakness.

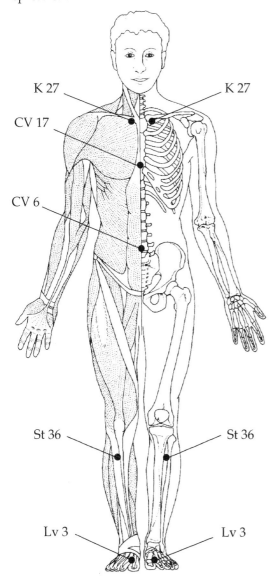

Three Mile Point (St 36)

Location: Four finger widths below the kneecap, one finger width to the outside of the shinbone. If you are on the correct spot, a muscle should flex as you move your foot up and down.

Benefits: Strengthens the whole body, especially the immune system; tones the muscles and aids digestion as well as relieves fatigue.

Bigger Stream (K 3)

Caution: This point should not be stimulated strongly after the third month of pregnancy.

Location: Midway between the inside of the anklebone and the Achilles tendon in the back of the ankle.

Benefits: Strengthens the immune system; relieves fatigue, swollen feet, and ankle pain.

Bigger Rushing (Lv 3)

Location: On the top of the foot, in the valley between the big toe and the second toe.

Benefits: Boosts the immune system; relieves fainting, eye fatigue, headaches, and hangovers.

Crooked Pond (LI 11)

Location: On the upper edge of the elbow crease.

Benefits: Relieves immune system weaknesses, fever, constipation, and elbow pain.

Outer Gate (TW 5)

Location: Two and one-half finger widths above the center of the wrist crease on the outside of the forearm midway between the two bones (ulna and radius).

Benefits: Relieves rheumatism, tendonitis, and wrist pain, and increases resistance to colds.

Joining the Valley (Hoku) (LI 4)

Caution: This point is forbidden for pregnant women because its stimulation can cause premature contractions in the uterus.

Location: In the webbing between the thumb and index finger at the highest spot of the muscle when the thumb and index finger are brought close together.

Benefits: Relieves arthritis, constipation, headaches, toothaches, shoulder pain, and labor pain.

Sea of Tranquility (CV 17)

Location: On the center of the breastbone three thumb widths up from the base of the bone.

Benefits: Relieves anxiety, anguish, and depression; boosts the immune system and regulates the thymus gland.

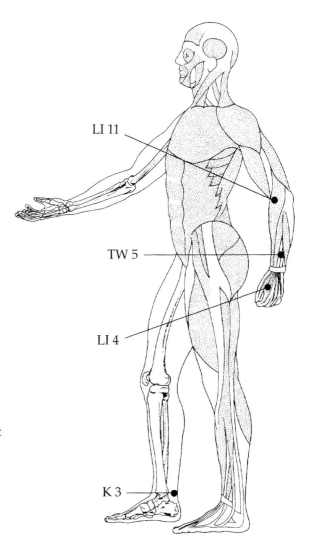

■ *You do not have to use all of these points. Using just one or two of them whenever you have a free hand can be effective.*

Potent Point Exercises

Sit comfortably for this routine and loosen your clothing if necessary.

Step 1

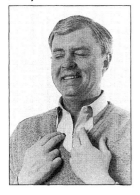

Firmly hold K 27: Place your middle fingers in the hollows directly below the protrusions of the collarbone just outside your upper breastbone. Breathe deeply as you hold for one minute.

Sit forward on the lip of your chair for the next exercise.

Step 2

Briskly rub B 23 and B 47: Place the backs of your hands against your lower back. Rub up and down briskly for one minute, creating heat from the friction. This self-massage will stimulate both lower back points.

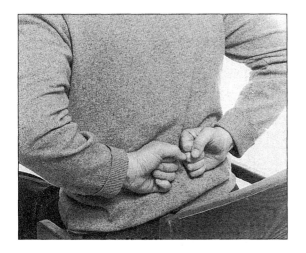

Sit back comfortably and continue.

Step 3

Firmly press CV 6: Place your fingertips in the center of your lower abdominal area, between your belly button and pubic bone.

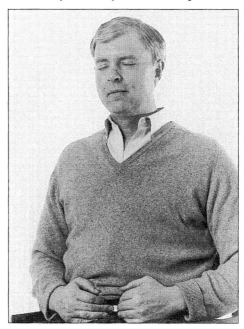

Gradually press one to two inches deep inside the lower abdomen. Close your eyes as you breathe deeply.

Step 4

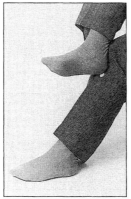

Briskly rub St 36: Place your right heel on the Three Mile point (St 36) of your left leg and briskly rub it up and down on the outside of your shinbone, just below your knee. After one minute, do the same on the other side.

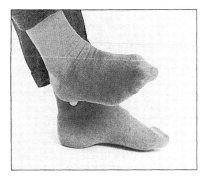

Step 5

Rub K 3 and then Lv 3: Place your right heel between your left inner anklebone and the Achilles tendon. After rubbing K 3 for thirty seconds, place your right heel in the juncture between the bones that attach to the large and

second toes to rub Lv 3 for thirty seconds. Then switch sides to stimulate these two points on your other foot for thirty seconds each.

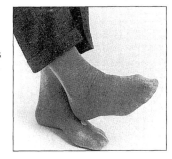

Step 6

Briskly rub LI 11: With your arms bent in front of you and your palms down, place the palm side of your right fist on top of the elbow crease of your left hand. Briskly rub over the elbow joint with your palm for thirty seconds, creating heat with the friction. Then do the same on the other arm.

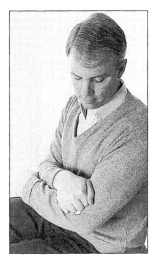

Step 7

Rub TW 5 and then LI 4: Make a fist with your right hand and place it on the outside of your forearm, two finger widths from your

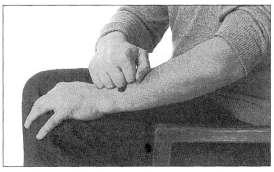

wrist crease. Briskly rub TW 5 for thirty seconds. Then place your right fist on the webbing between the thumb and index finger of your left hand. Use your knuckles to briskly rub the Hoku point for thirty seconds. Switch arms and stimulate these two points on the other side.

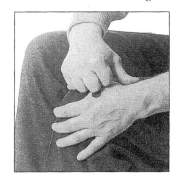

Step 8

Repeat steps 1 and 2: This will further boost your immune system.

Step 9

Press CV 17: Keeping your palms together, place the back of your thumbs firmly against your breastbone to press CV 17, at the level of your heart. Continue to keep your eyes closed and concentrate on breathing slow, even, deep breaths into your heart to completely dispel any anxiety. Use the following exercise.

A Breathing Exercise for the Immune System

Focus on breathing deeply for two more minutes. Gently control your respiratory system, making each breath grow longer and deeper than the last one. Breathe out any tensions you feel restricting your lungs from moving fully and naturally. Feel your mind clear with each breath. Notice the resistance your mind creates: the worries and judgments it comes up against. Take several deep breaths and dissolve these barriers. Breathe deeply and gently; remember, you are breathing in life itself.

Hold the breath at the top of the exhalation for a moment, feeling its fullness. Then exhale smoothly, letting your hands drift down into your lap, and relax, feeling the vitality of the breath circulate throughout your body.

Additional Points for Boosting the Immune System

For illustrations of related points for boosting the immune system, see chapter 11, "Colds and Flu"; and chapter 10, "Chronic Fatigue Syndrome."

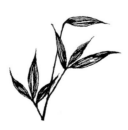

24
IMPOTENCY AND SEXUAL PROBLEMS

*L*ifestyle habits and stressful situations can affect sexual potency. Depending on how we live and how we respond to life circumstances, we can either build or deplete our energy reserves, directly affecting our potency. Emotional imbalances can affect potency, too, whether they occur in intimate relationships or with other circumstances of your life.

A sexual relationship is one of the most intimate of situations and can cause feelings of vulnerability. For many people, sex is an expression of love and tenderness. But inner pressures, such as fear, insecurity, and performance anxiety, can cause tensions that interfere with the pleasures of sex. For men, premature ejaculation can often be the result of anxiety caused by pressure to perform. In women, emotional stress and pressure can be expressed by vaginal infections, menstrual cramps, lack of sexual desire, or other problems related to the genitals.

If you suffer from impotency, first consult with your doctor to see if you have an underlying organic or physical condition. Other contributing causes of impotency can be excessive alcohol or drugs, diabetes, or nerve damage. Impotency is also a frequent side effect of some medications.

Chinese medicine traditionally describes potency and sexual activity as governed by the kidneys. A lifestyle and diet that stresses the kidneys and generally weakens your health can also cause impotency by depleting the kidneys' energy. The consumption of alcohol, drugs, white sugar, and excess fluids; exposure to cold; overall fatigue; and chronic lower-back problems can all contribute to impotency.

Ways to Strengthen Potency

There are many ways to recharge the kidneys and improve your sex life. Emotional expressions that encourage openness, trust, communication, and the willingness to let go of expectations and judgments can greatly ease interpersonal problems that may be affecting your enjoyment of sex. You can strengthen potency by improving physical health, including getting regular exercise and eating a balanced diet.

Diet

A common Oriental folk remedy uses beans to benefit the reproductive organs:

Azuki beans are excellent for kidney disorders. Black beans are good for the sexual organs, for example in cases of irregular menstruation, barrenness, and a lack of sexual appetite.[35]

Eating a mixture of three parts grain to one part beans not only combines all the essential amino acids to make a complete protein, but also strengthens the sexual-reproductive systems in both men and women. According to traditional Chinese medicine, an excess of sugar can imbalance the spleen, pancreas, and liver, which taxes the kidneys. Avoiding sugar and eating a balanced diet of whole, fresh foods (apples are especially beneficial) contribute to overall good health and a high level of energy, both of which are valuable components of sexual potency.

---

[35] Muramoto, Noboru, *Healing Ourselves* (New York: Avon Books, 1983), 72.

Potent Points for Impotency

Chronic muscular tension in the pelvic region can contribute to impotency, lack of sexual drive, weak erection, premature ejaculation, vaginal infections, and menstrual cramps. When the muscles of the pelvic area are chronically tense, circulation to the genitals is decreased. Various factors, such as restrictive clothing, poor posture, lack of exercise, chest and shoulder tension, emotional stress, and frustration often contribute to pelvic and abdominal tension. For potency and sexual sensations to be as full as possible, the pelvic area must be flexible. When tension is released, it is possible to experience a greater depth of feeling; when the pelvic area is free and open, pleasurable sensations and the experience of orgasm can deepen.

Pressing acupressure points in the pelvic and abdominal areas increases the flow of blood and sensory impulses through the reproductive organs. There are also acupressure points related to the kidneys that aid potency. Because acupressure increases circulation and works to build overall health, it also fortifies the body's sexual functions. The points in the lower back and the base of the spine (the sacrum), for example, relieve menstrual disorders and irregularities in the prostate gland and the bladder. The following points strengthen the male and female sexual-reproductive systems.

Potent Points for Relieving Impotency

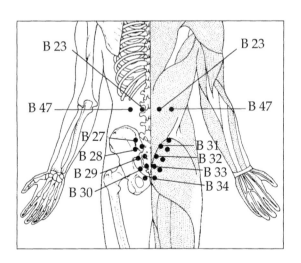

B 23

B 23

B 47

B 47

B 27

B 31

B 28

B 32

B 29

B 33

B 30

B 34

Sea of Vitality (B 23 and B 47)

Caution: Do not press on disintegrating discs or fractured or broken bones. If you have a weak back, a few minutes of stationary, light touching instead of pressure can be very healing. See your doctor first if you have any questions or need medical advice.

Location: On the lower back (between the second and third lumbar vertebrae) two to four finger widths away from the spine at waist level, in line with the belly button.

Benefits: Relieves lower-back aches, fatigue, sexual-reproductive problems, impotency, and premature ejaculation.

Point Number	Benefits and Uses
B 27 & B 28	Relieves hip pain (especially in the sacroiliac joint), sexual-reproductive problems, and retention of urine
B 29 & B 30	Relieves impotency, lumbago, sacral pain, and sciatica
B 31 & B 32	Relieves lumbago and impotency
B 33 & B 34	Relieves sterility, irregular vaginal discharge, and genital pain

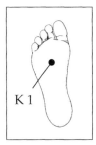 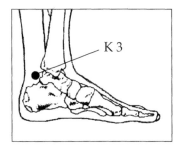

Bubbling Springs (K 1)

Location: On the center of the sole of the foot, at the base of the ball of the foot, between the two pads.

Benefits: Relieves hot flashes as well as impotency.

Bigger Stream (K 3)

Caution: This point should not be stimulated strongly after the third month of pregnancy.

Location: Midway between the inside anklebone and the Achilles tendon in the back of the ankle.

Benefits: Relieves sexual tensions, semen leakage, menstrual irregularity, swollen feet, ankle pain, and fatigue.

Three Mile Point (St 36)

Location: Four finger widths below the kneecap, one finger width on the outside of the shinbone. If you are on the correct spot, a muscle should flex as you move your foot up and down.

Benefits: Strengthens the whole body, especially the muscles, and aids the sexual-reproductive systems. It normally takes months of daily practice to relieve impotency.

Gate Origin (CV 4)

Location: Four finger widths directly below the belly button.

Benefits: Relieves impotency, uroreproductive problems, irregular vaginal discharge, irregular menstrual periods, and urinary incontinence.

Sacral Points (B 27-B 34)

The acupressure points on the base of the spine (see illustration) also help relieve menstrual cramps and lower back pain. Steady, firm pressure on these sacral points — which are directly related to the reproductive system — can help impotency.

Sea of Energy (CV 6)

Location: Three finger widths directly below the belly button.

Benefits: Relieves uroreproductive problems, irregular vaginal discharge, irregular periods, and impotency. Also used for strengthening the reproductive system.

Rushing Door (Sp 12)
Mansion Cottage (Sp 13)

These two points are especially effective for releasing menstrual discomforts.

Location: Both points are in the pelvic area in the middle of the crease where the leg joins the trunk of the body.

Benefits: These points are particularly good for relieving impotency, menstrual cramps, and abdominal discomfort.

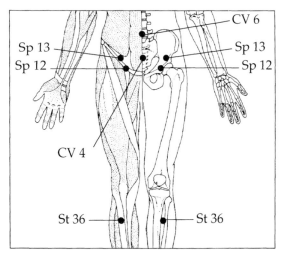

■ *You do not have to use all of these points. Using just one or two of them whenever you have a free hand can be effective.*

Potent Point Exercises

Sit comfortably during the first three steps of this routine.

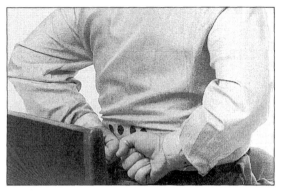

Step 1

Rub B 47 and B 23: Use the backs of your hands to rub your lower back points briskly up and down, creating heat from the friction for one minute. Next, firmly press B 47 (on the outer edge of the large vertical muscles that run alongside the spine) in toward the center of the vertebrae for one minute. Then stimulate B 23 by pressing the top of the large vertical muscles about two finger widths away from the spine. Use either your thumbs or your fingers to stimulate one side at a time or both sides at once, holding for at least one minute.

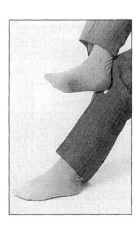

Step 2

Briskly rub St 36: Place your right heel on the left St 36 point, outside of your leg below your knee. Use your heel to briskly rub this point for thirty seconds. Then switch sides and do the same on your opposite leg.

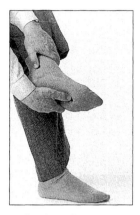

Step 3

Press K 3 with K 1: Comfortably position your left foot on your right thigh. Then place your left thumb on K 3 between the Achilles tendon and the inside anklebone, angling your pressure in the direction underneath your inner anklebone. Use your right thumb to press K 1 in the center of the sole of the foot. Hold these points firmly for one minute as you concentrate on breathing deeply. Then switch to hold these points on your other foot for one minute.

Lie down comfortably on your back with your knees bent, feet flat on the floor.

Step 4

Press CV 4 and CV 6: Place the fingertips of one hand just above the center of your pubic bone on CV 4 and the fingers of your other hand just above that, between your belly button and pubic bone on CV 6. Close your eyes and breathe deeply as you apply firm

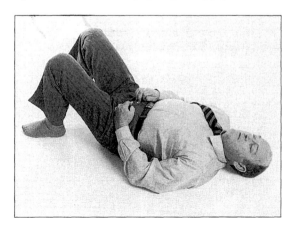

pressure one to two inches deep into the abdomen into these important potency points for one to two minutes. Carefully using a hot water bottle on these points can also be very beneficial.[36]

Step 5

Hold or lie on Sp 12 and Sp 13: Use all of your fingertips to press directly on the thick, ropy ligament located in the center of the leg crease at the top and front of your thigh for one minute. While pressing these points, you'll be able to feel a strong pulsation from a large artery that runs between these points and your genitals.[37]

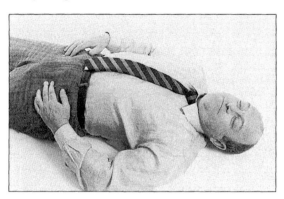

Step 6

Press points B 27-B 34: While still lying on your back with your knees bent, feet flat on the floor, lift your pelvis up and place your hands one on top of the other, palms down, under the sacrum at the base of your spine. Reposition your hands so that the fingers of one hand are crossed on top of the fingers of the other. Slowly lower your pelvis onto your hands. Then let your knees sway from side to side for one minute as you breathe deeply into your belly. An optional move is to bring your feet several inches off the ground and move your knees in a large, slow circular motion.

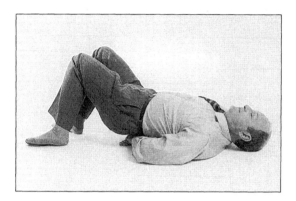

[36] Heat on these lower abdominal points fortifies the sexual-reproductive system. Try using hot compresses such as a hot water bottle, a heating pad, or carefully using a hand-held hair dryer to gently warm these potent points for a few minutes.
[37] A method for stimulating these groin points more deeply is to lie flat on your abdomen, placing your fists in your groin. Bring your forehead or your chin to the floor and your feet together. Then inhale and raise your feet up with your thighs off the ground. This will put pressure on these potency points. Begin long, deep breathing with your legs up for thirty seconds. Then let your legs come down and your hands relax at your sides. Adjust your body comfortably and completely relax for one minute.

Step 7

Repeat step 4: Press CV 4 and CV 6 once again for one minute, breathing deeply to achieve greater potency.

Additional Points for Relieving Impotency

For illustrations of other related points for relieving impotency, see chapter 9, "Backache and Sciatica"; and chapter 23, "Immune System Boosting."

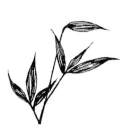

25

INSOMNIA

*I*nsomniacs are unable to sleep continuously and peacefully for a period of four to eight hours. Sleep that is prematurely ended or interrupted often leads to irritability and, eventually, ill health. According to Keith Kenyon, M.D., everyone will suffer from insomnia at one time or another. Because it can be an agonizing experience and because sleeping pills are unhealthy and only increase sleep problems, acupressure can be a valuable resource.[38]

Stress, pain, grief, and anxiety can exacerbate sleeping disorders. Peace of mind is essential to falling asleep. If pain is causing insomnia, you must relieve the pain to promote a relaxed, beneficial sleep.

According to traditional Chinese medicine, an uneven distribution of energy can also cause insomnia. In such cases, certain meridians (the energy pathways that connect acupressure points) become overloaded, while others become blocked. By pressing certain points, you can correct this energy imbalance. A regimen that incorporates acupressure, a proper diet, and the following relaxation techniques is highly effective for relieving insomnia.

Many of my acupressure students have had great success in helping their spouses or children overcome insomnia. They consistently report that in a one-hour session, their clients often relax so deeply that they fall asleep as their points are being pressed. Although this relaxation is immediate, a couple of months of regular self-acupressure is usually necessary to change your overall sleeping pattern.

Basically, three sets of points are used: the points underneath the base of the skull, those between the shoulder blades, and the points on both the ankles. As a result, people report that they not only sleep more deeply without waking, they also tend to feel more alert and have greater energy the following day.

A client of mine, Nancy, who had recently gone through a divorce and was caring for two teenage children, suffered from insomnia. She had not slept well for three months and was exhausted. I showed her how to work on her neck, chest, and ankle points. I also told her to drink fresh ginger tea with a little honey instead of the three cups of coffee she drank each day. When I called Nancy after ten days, she told me her mental outlook had improved and she was sleeping well.

Diet

Foods that are high in saturated fat and cholesterol increase blood cholesterol levels. The blood carries these fatty deposits, which attach to the walls of the blood vessels, narrowing the passageways. The heart is forced to work harder to pump the blood through narrower vessels. Overconsumption of fat and cholesterol is a major contributing factor to coronary heart disease and certain kinds of cancer. In traditional Chinese medicine, the heart also is believed to affect one's ability to sleep.

---

[38] Keith Kenyon, M.D., *Do-It-Yourself Acupuncture Without Needles* (New York: Arco Publishing, 1977), 92.

Natural Ways to Induce Sleep

- **Stretching:** Stretch and exaggerate a few yawns to help relax your body and prepare it for sleep.

- **Eye Exercises:** While sitting or lying down in bed, look up as far as you can, and then slowly move your eyes in a circle around the periphery of your vision three times. Repeat the eye rotation in the opposite direction three more times.

- **Deep Breathing:** Concentrate on breathing deeply into your belly when you are in bed and trying to get to sleep; this can reduce tension in your body. Tension and stress strongly contribute to an inability to fall asleep and stay asleep.

- **Deep Relaxation:** Lie on your back with your eyes closed. Starting with your toes, mentally tell each part of your body to relax as you take long, slow, deep breaths.

Potent Points for Relieving Insomnia

The acupressure points on the heel have traditionally been used for relieving and preventing insomnia. The point on the inside of the heel is called Joyful Sleep; the one on the outside of the heel is called Calm Sleep. Massaging and pressing these points together on both sides of the heel enables the body to relax deeply and promote sleep. This is a technique you can teach your child.

According to Chinese health care, insomnia is also related to the heart and pericardium meridians. If you have a blockage in either of these meridians, you may have difficulty sleeping. Traditionally, the points called Spirit Gate (located on the inside of the wrist, below the little finger) and Inner Gate (located on the center of the inner wrist, two finger widths above the wrist crease) have been used for insomnia. These points help balance and calm the heart, alleviate anxiety, and enable you to sleep soundly at night.

Vital Diaphragm (B 38)

Location: Between the shoulder blades and the spine at heart level.

Benefits: This upper back point relieves insomnia, and calms high emotions such as anxiety, which can inhibit sleep.

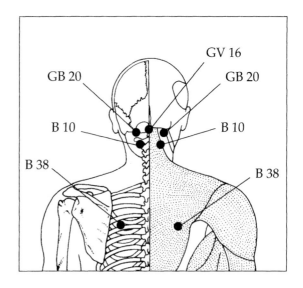

Inner Gate (P 6)

Location: In the middle of the inner side of the forearm, two and one-half finger widths from the wrist crease.

Benefits: Relieves insomnia and several other common complaints that can keep one from sleeping, such as anxiety, palpitations, nausea, and indigestion.

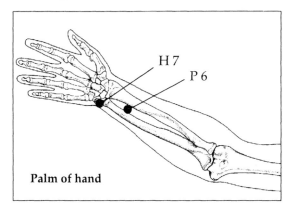

Palm of hand

Spirit Gate (H 7)

Location: On the inside of the wrist crease, in line with the little finger.

Benefits: Relieves anxiety, cold sweats, and insomnia due to overexcitement.

Heavenly Pillar (B 10)

Location: One-half inch below the base of the skull on the ropy muscles located one-half inch outward from the spine.

Benefits: Relieves insomnia, stress, burnout, and exhaustion.

Wind Mansion (GV 16)

Location: In the center of the back of the head in a large hollow under the base of the skull.

Benefits: Relieves insomnia as well as mental stress.

■ *You do not have to use all of these points. Using just one or two of them whenever you have a free hand can be effective.*

Gates of Consciousness (GB 20)

Location: Below the base of the skull, in the hollow between the two large vertical neck muscles, two to three inches apart depending on the size of the head.

Benefits: Relieves arthritis, headaches, and neck pain that causes insomnia.

Third Eye Point (GV 24.5)

Location: Directly between the eyebrows, in the indentation where the bridge of the nose meets the forehead.

Benefits: Relaxes the central nervous system for relieving anxiety and insomnia.

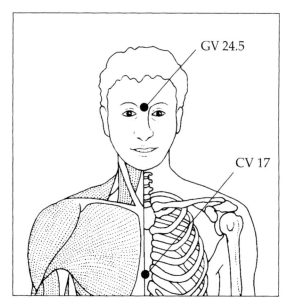

Sea of Tranquility (CV 17)

Location: On the center of the breastbone three thumb widths up from the base of the bone.

Benefits: Relieves nervousness, chest congestion, and the anxiety that causes insomnia.

133

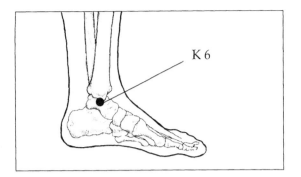

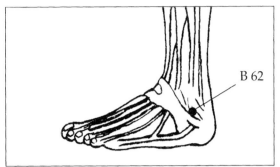

Joyful Sleep (K 6)

Location: Directly below the inside of the anklebone in a slight indentation.

Benefits: Relieves insomnia, heel and ankle pain, hypertension and anxiety.

Calm Sleep (B 62)

Location: In the first indentation directly below the outer anklebone.

Benefits: Relieves insomnia and the back pain that makes it difficult to sleep.

Potent Point Exercises

The following routine is most effective when done lying down. However, you can also practice all these acupressure techniques (except step 1) sitting comfortably.

Step 1

Use tennis balls to press B 38: Lie down on two tennis balls, placing them between your shoulder blades. Close your eyes and breathe deeply for one minute.

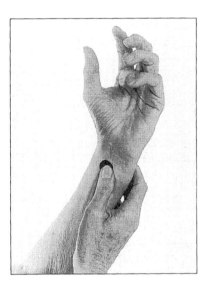

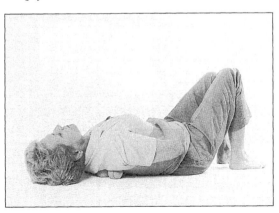

Step 2

Press P 6: Place your right thumb on the inside of your left wrist with your fingers directly behind, two and one-half finger widths below the wrist crease. Press firmly for one minute. Then press the point on your other wrist.

Step 3

Hold H 7: Place your thumb or the fingers of your right hand on the inside wrist crease of your left hand. Press into the H 7 point, the hollow in the crease directly below your little finger. After holding for one minute, switch sides to hold the point on your right wrist.

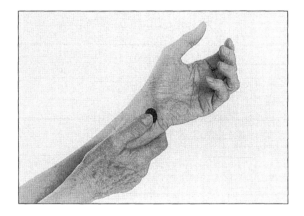

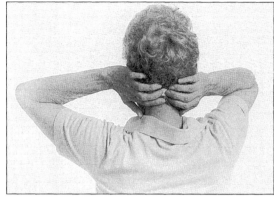

Step 5

Press GV 16: Place your middle fingers in the large hollow at the center of the base of your skull. Close your eyes, slowly tilt your head back and breathe deeply as you press firmly into this hollow area for one to two minutes. Induce yawning while holding this point if you're trying to get to sleep.

Step 4

Firmly press B 10: Curve your fingers, placing your fingertips on the thick, ropy muscles on the back of your neck. Apply firm pressure as you breathe deeply for one minute.

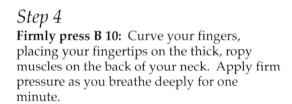

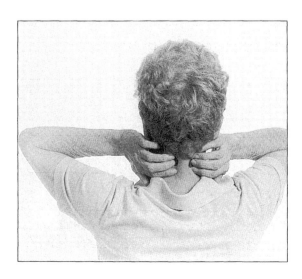

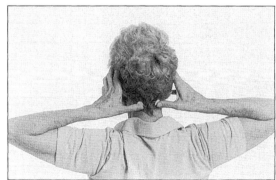

Step 6

Press up into GB 20: Use your thumbs to gradually press underneath the base of your skull, two to three inches apart depending on the size of your head. Keeping your eyes closed, slowly tilt your head back as you use your thumbs to firmly press up and underneath your skull for one to two minutes or until you feel a regular, even pulse on both sides.

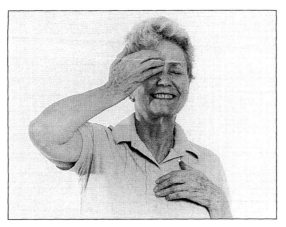

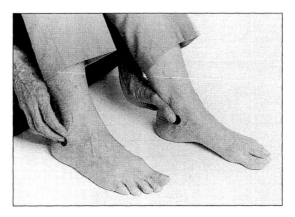

Step 7

Hold GV 24.5 along with CV 17: Place your right middle fingertip in between your eyebrows in the indentation between the bridge of your nose and your forehead. Position the fingertips of your left hand on CV 17, in the indentations of your breastbone at the level of your heart. Close your eyes and breathe deeply for one minute.

Step 8

Hold K 6 with B 62: Use your thumbs to hold the K 6 points on the inside of each ankle in an indentation directly below the inner ankle-bone. Position your fingertips directly across from your thumb to press B 62, which is located directly below the outer anklebone. Hold these points for one minute as you breathe deeply, to relieve insomnia.

Additional Points for Relieving Insomnia

For illustrations of other related points for relieving insomnia, see chapter 6, "Anxiety and Nervousness"; chapter 8, "Asthma and Breathing Difficulties"; and chapter 35, "Pain."

26

IRRITABILITY, FRUSTRATION, AND DEALING WITH CHANGE

*E*verything happens at its own pace. Every flower and tree matures at its own rhythm. People also have distinctly individual patterns of change and development. When we are irritated or frustrated, however, we are not flowing with what's happening in our lives, but rather are pushing or resisting something. The key to dissolving frustration is to open our perspective, and accept our limitations in controlling a situation.

> *When one encounters an obstruction...*
> *one should not strive blindly to go ahead,*
> *for this only leads to complications. The*
> *correct thing is, on the contrary, to retreat*
> *for the time being, not in order to give up*
> *the struggle, but to await the right moment*
> *for action. Ordinarily it is best to go*
> *around an obstruction and try to overcome*
> *it along the line of least resistance.[39]*

Next time you become frustrated, step aside from your situation for a moment and observe what's going on. What is the obstacle involved? Examine it and see what it means to you, how it represents ways you hold yourself back ("I can't," "I don't want to," "I'm not good, smart, talented, or rich enough," "It's too hard," etc.).

Decide to perceive the obstacle as only one aspect of your life. Think of it as a choice you have made, something you have decided to deal with instead of seeing yourself as stuck in the situation, overwhelmed by your frustration. Letting go of anger or resentment

toward the situation allows other possibilities to emerge.

Sometimes you may simply want to accept the obstacle and "put it on hold" for the time being; at other times you may choose to work through it. Follow your intuition, and do what feels right.

Linda, one of my long-time friends, was facing problems with Danny, her teenage son. He had recently started hanging out with kids who were into alcohol. She was not only concerned with her son's safety, but was frustrated that his lack of responsibility was jeopardizing her own plans. Danny, who had promised to be home that afternoon, was more than forty-five minutes late and Linda was getting ready to take a trip. Instead of holding on to her expectations and anxiety, Linda spent a half hour doing the acupressure exercises in this chapter together with deep breathing exercises. By the time Danny arrived home with his excuses about rush-hour traffic, Linda's perspective on the situation had opened up, and she was able to set up a concrete agreement with her son that enabled her to go out of town with peace of mind.

We are continuously being tested. If you can perceive a frustrating experience as something you willingly take on, you can transform it from an impediment to an opportunity for growth.

Areas of Muscular Tension

Frustration and irritation collect mainly in the shoulders, neck, solar plexus, and hips. Acupressure in these areas can help release

---

[39] Wilhelm/Baynes, *The I Ching*, or *The Book of Changes*, (Princeton: Princeton University Press, 1967), 152.

these harmful emotions and circumvent unhealthy impulses such as smoking, drinking, and overeating, which often stem from emotional imbalance. (The following points are described in detail later in this chapter.)

Shoulders: Potent point GB 21 releases tension in the shoulders and helps you deal with irritability.

The solar plexus: This area is related to your personal power and self-image. Tensions here can result from feeling insecure about yourself and your abilities, or, conversely, from a fear of your own power and of being recognized (and punished) for it — a fear of success. Potent point CV 12, located in the pit of the stomach, helps you release deep frustrations that relate to some aspect of your life or yourself that you are repressing or restricting.

Neck: Tension in the neck is often associated with anger. Frustrations can literally become a "pain in the neck." Repressing your anger, which seems to jam your feelings down your throat instead of expressing what you really want to say, creates neck tension. Potent point GB 20, underneath the base of the skull, is effective for releasing neck pain and tension.

Hips: The hips are also associated with frustration and irritation. When people stand with their hands on their hips, they are often feeling frustrated or irritated. Not coincidentally, they are also instinctively holding

acupressure points that can relieve that frustration. Potent points GB 30 and B 48 in the pelvic region help release the muscular tensions at the very core of irritations and pent-up frustrations.

The opposite of frustration and irritation is well-being, the sense of being "in the flow" of things, a sense of harmony and aliveness. The acupressure points described in this chapter work on the areas where tensions related to irritability and frustration tend to collect. The Third Eye Point (GV 24.5) and the Sea of Tranquility (CV 17), which calm and relax the spirit, also enable us to envision and create new insights. You can teach these points to your child to help him or her manage frustration and irritability.

I use these points every day. I hold CV 17 on the center of my breastbone when I feel frustrated, irritated, or tense. This point releases the tightness in my chest and enables me to take deep breaths, which have an instant calming effect.

I also use the Third Eye Point in a number of ways to enhance my life. You can collect your thoughts and revitalize yourself by closing your eyes and rolling them upward as you lift your eyebrows and lightly touch the point between your brows. Take a few deep breaths and concentrate all of your attention on this point. This focusing of your mind and body can give you the brief relaxation and open space you may need to rejuvenate your energy for dealing with change.

Potent Points for Relieving Frustration and Irritation

Shoulder Well (GB 21)

Caution: Pregnant women should press this point lightly.

Location: On the highest point of the shoulder muscle midway between the outer tip of the shoulder and the spine.

Benefits: Relieves frustration, irritability, fatigue, shoulder tension, and nervousness.

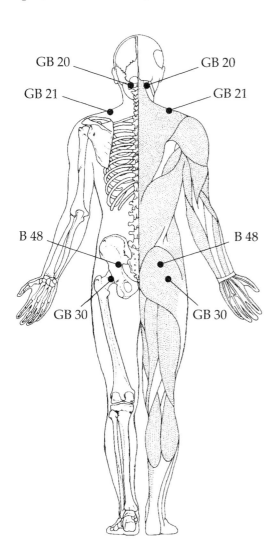

Center of Power (CV 12)

Caution: Do not hold this point deeply if you have a serious illness. (See caution on page 9.) It is best not to hold this point for more than two minutes and to use it only on a fairly empty stomach.

Location: On the center (midline) of the body, midway between the base of the breastbone and the belly button.

Benefits: Relieves frustration, stomach pains, abdominal spasms, indigestion, emotional stress, and headaches.

Womb and Vitals (B 48)

Location: Two finger widths outside the widest portion of the sacrum at the level of the hipbone.

Benefits: Relieves frustration, irritation, pelvic tension, sciatica, lower-back aches, and hip pain.

Jumping Circle (GB 30)

Location: In the center of each buttock, in back of the most prominent part of the upper thigh bone.

Benefits: Relieves frustration, irritation, hip pain, sciatica, lower back pain, and rheumatism.

Letting Go (Lu 1)

Location: On the outer part of the upper chest, four finger widths up from the armpit crease and one finger width inward.

Benefits: Relieves breathing difficulties, chest tension and congestion, emotional tensions, coughing, asthma, and skin disorders.

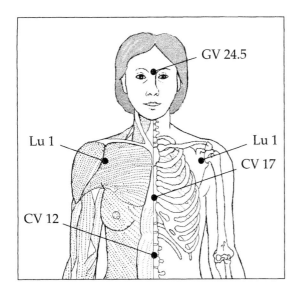

Third Eye Point (GV 24.5)

Location: Directly between your eyebrows, in the indentation where the bridge of the nose meets the forehead.

Benefits: Good for spiritual and emotional imbalances, and relieves hay fever, headaches, indigestion, ulcer pain, and eyestrain.

Sea of Tranquility (CV 17)

Location: On the center of the breastbone three thumb widths up from the base of the bone.

Benefits: Relieves nervousness, anxiety, frustration, irritability, chest congestion, insomnia, and depression.

◼ *You do not have to use all of these points. Using just one or two of them whenever you have a free hand can be effective.*

Gates of Consciousness (GB 20)

Location: Below the base of the skull, in the hollow between the two large vertical neck muscles, two to three inches apart depending on the size of the head.

Benefits: Relieves irritability, headaches, dizziness, arthritis, neck pain, injuries, trauma, shock, and hypertension.

Potent Point Exercises

Sit comfortably and breathe deeply as you hold each of the following points.

Step 1

Firmly press GB 21: Curve your fingers, placing your fingertips on the tops of your shoulders, and press directly into the shoulder tension. Bring your head up and back as you inhale, and exhale as you lower your head downward. Continue this easy movement of your head with long, deep breathing as you hold these shoulder points for one minute.

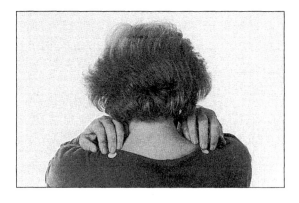

Step 2

Press CV 12: Place the fingertips of both hands between your belly button and the base of your breast-bone. Gradually apply firm pressure in and upward, leaning your upper body forward, to press deeply into the pit of your stomach as you breathe deeply for one minute.

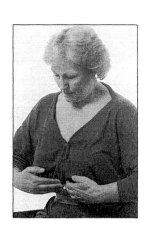

Lean forward on to the lip of your chair or stand to work on the next two points. If you have at least ten more minutes and can lie down comfortably on a carpeted floor, then substitute the "Frustration Release Exercise" that follows these Potent Point Exercises for step 3. That exercise will enable you to stimulate these potent points with greater strength and depth.

Step 3

Press B 48 and GB 30: Place your thumbs on the muscles of your buttocks to press B 48 just below your lower back. Take several long, slow, deep breaths as you firmly press inward (toward the center of your pelvis) for one minute. Then make fists and slide them one inch down and one inch outward to press GB 30 for another minute.

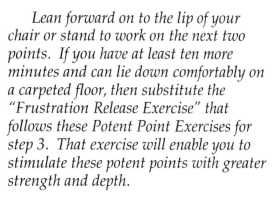

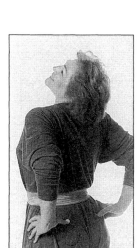

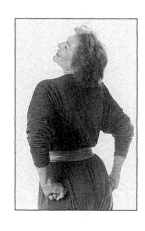

Sit comfortably to complete this self-acupressure treatment.

Step 4

Press Lu 1: Place your thumbs on the upper, outer portion of your chest, feeling for tension there. Make firm contact with the muscles

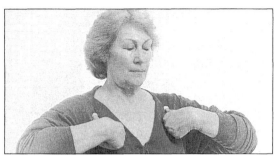

located four finger widths up and one finger width inward from your armpit. Close your eyes and concentrate on breathing deeply as you hold these chest points for one minute to relieve any irritability or frustration.

Step 5

Firmly press up into GB 20: Place your thumbs underneath the base of your skull into the indentations that lie two to three inches apart. Slowly tilt your head back as you press

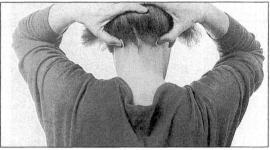

up and underneath your skull, concentrating on breathing deeply for one minute or until you feel a regular, even pulse on both sides. Then very slowly release the pressure.

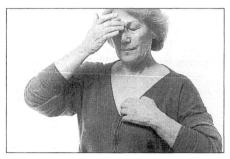

Step 6

Hold the GV 24.5 with CV 17: Gently place your right middle fingertip in between your eyebrows on GV 24.5 in the slight indentation just above the bridge of your nose. Use the fingertips of your left hand to hold CV 17 in the indentations in the center of your breastbone. Close your eyes and breathe deeply into these points for at least a minute.

Frustration Release Exercise

Lie down comfortably on your back.
1. Place your hands or fists, palms down, under your buttocks.

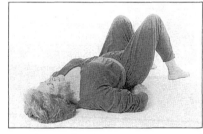

2. Bend your knees and place your feet comfortably apart.
3. Move your knees from side to side; your knuckles should be pressing into your buttocks muscles in this position.
4. Inhale as the knees come back to center.
5. Continue for one or two minutes, alternating sides.
6. Relax on your back with your eyes closed as you take long, deep breaths.

Additional Points for Relieving Irritability and Frustration

For illustrations of other related points for relieving irritability and frustration, see chapter 6, "Anxiety and Nervousness"; and chapter 14, "Depression and Emotional Balancing."

27

JAW PROBLEMS
(TMJ PROBLEMS)

$\mathcal{M}$any people unconsciously clench or grind their teeth when they sleep. This causes "dental stress," which damages the teeth, as well as causing TMJ problems. The TMJ (temporomandibular joint) connects the jaw bone to the cranium, just below and beside the ear. You can find the joint by pressing your fingers firmly into the side of your cheek near the ear and moving your jaw up and down. Sufferers of rheumatoid arthritis often experience problems in this area — inflammation, spasms, swelling, and pain. Acupressure along with facial exercises are an excellent way to eliminate TMJ pain and discomfort.

Some people have difficulty opening their mouth widely. Sometimes a simple movement, for example trying to get your mouth around a thick sandwich, can cause the jaw muscles to spasm. To relieve this cramping, hold the Jaw Chariot point (St 6), applying gradual, firm pressure directly on the jaw spasm for two to three minutes.

Try the following jaw exercise to enable you to open your mouth wider and prevent spasms. First, look into a mirror to see how wide you can open your mouth. Then bite down firmly onto a wooden clothespin, chopstick, or kitchen spoon handle for five seconds. Release your bite and relax your jaw. Repeat this several times as you take long, deep breaths.

TMJ and Dental Stress
(Clenching the Teeth)

I used to wake up many mornings with my teeth tightly clenched together. My dentist told me I had TMJ syndrome. He concluded that I had been grinding my teeth in my sleep. He explained that the grinding puts stress on the jawbone so that it will eventually wear away. As it deteriorates, the teeth loosen and eventually have to be pulled. "If you continue to clench your teeth, you'll end up having to wear dentures," he said. I took his diagnosis seriously and decided to create an acupressure routine for treating my TMJ problem.

I used only one bilateral acupressure point (St 6), pressing with firm, prolonged pressure for two minutes three times daily. At the end of one month, the intermittent aching in my jaw had disappeared.

Now it has been years since I began using acupressure to deal with my TMJ problem and I rarely wake up clenching my jaws. Occasionally, I find that my jaws are tense. When I give myself acupressure using the St 6 point, pressing with firm, prolonged pressure for just a few minutes, the tension eases. I still tend to collect stress in the jaws, and I often find myself naturally pressing this jaw point to manage the dental stress, especially in bed before going to sleep.

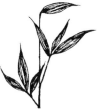

Potent Points for Relieving Jaw Problems

Jaw Chariot (St 6)

Location: Between the upper and lower jaw, on the (masseter) muscle that bulges when the back teeth are clenched.

Benefits: Relieves jaw pain and spasms, TMJ problems, lockjaw, dental neuralgia, and toothaches.

Wind Screen (TW 17)

Location: In the indentation underneath the earlobe.

Benefits: Relieves ear pain, facial paralysis, facial spasms, jaw pain, damp and itchy ears, throat swelling, mumps, and toothaches.

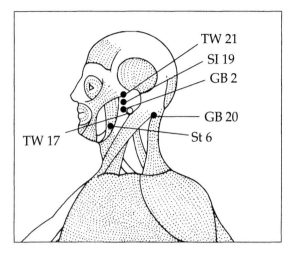

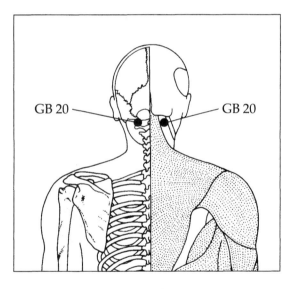

■ *You do not have to use all of these points. Using just one or two of them whenever you have a free hand can be effective.*

Listening Place (SI 19)
Ear Gate (TW 21)
Reunion of Hearing (GB 2)

Location: SI 19 is directly in front of the ear hole in a depression that enlarges when the mouth is open. TW 21 is one-half inch above this point; GB 2 is one-half inch below SI 19.

Benefits: Relieves jaw pain and the following head pains: earaches, pressure inside the ear, TMJ problems, toothaches, and headaches.

Gates of Consciousness (GB 20)

Location: Below the base of the skull, in the hollows two to three inches apart depending on the size of the head.

Benefits: Relieves jaw pain, and other related problems such as headaches, stiff necks, and neck pain.

Potent Point Exercises

If you regularly practice the following self-acupressure routine once or twice a day, you can relax your jaw muscles, maintain your full range of motion in this joint, release chronic tension, and prevent further jaw problems.

Step 1

Firmly press St 6 in two ways: First place the heel of your hand between your upper and lower jaws in front of the ear lobe, and gradually apply firm pressure. You should feel a muscle pop out when you clench your molars together. Press directly on the jaw muscle with your teeth slightly apart, breathing deeply, for one minute. Move your jaw left and right, taking a few more deep breaths.

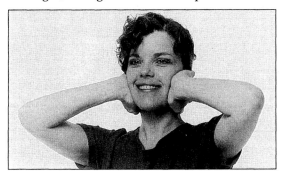

Now place your fingertips on the same jaw muscles to firmly press St 6 for another minute as you breathe deeply. Then gradually increase the pressure on the jaw muscle using your middle fingertips (with your index and ring fingertips close beside) to create a mild pain that is tolerable. Take long deep breaths into the pain with your

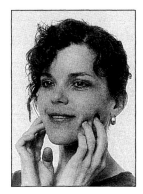

eyes closed in order to release any remaining tension in your jaw muscles. End with thirty seconds of light pressure as you continue to breathe deeply, feeling for a pulsation in your fingertips. The pulse indicates that healing energy is circulating through your jaw.

Step 2

Lightly press TW 17: Place your middle fingers underneath your earlobes and gradually apply light pressure on TW 17 into the

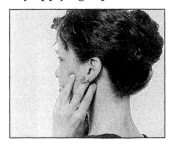

indentations behind your jawbone. These acupressure points are often very tender. Hold for one minute as you take long, deep breaths.

Step 3

Press SI 19, TW 21, and GB 2: Place your middle fingertips on SI 19 in front of your ear openings in the indentations that will expand when you open your mouth. Then place your

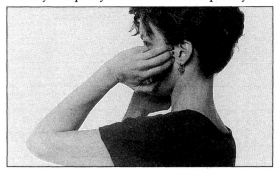

index and ring fingertips on either side of your middle fingers, pressing into the hollows between the bones. Concentrate on applying firm pressure for one minute on the lower of the three points (GB 2), because it is an important TMJ point for healing the jaw.

Step 4

Repeat step 1: Spend two more minutes firmly pressing St 6 as you breathe deeply.

Step 5

Relax as you press GB 20: Place your thumbs underneath the base of your skull in the indentations that lie two to three inches apart from the center, depending on the size of your head. Slowly tilt your head back, pressing up and underneath your skull as you continue to take long, slow, deep breaths. Hold these points for two minutes or until you feel a regular, even pulse on both sides. Then very slowly release the pressure.

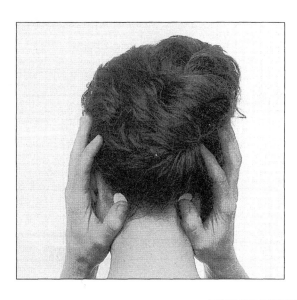

Additional Points for Relieving Jaw Pain

For illustrations of related points for relieving jaw pain, see chapter 16, "Earaches"; chapter 20, "Headaches and Migraines"; and chapter 41, "Toothaches."

Self-Acupressure Facial Massage

The following self-acupressure facial massage can be practiced after this TMJ relief point sequence or by itself to relieve jaw problems and enhance overall well-being.

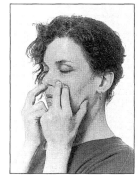

1. Use the tips of your middle fingers to massage slowly from the base of the nose between the eyes down to the sides of the nostrils several times.

2. Place your fingertips firmly on your jaw muscles (the muscles that contract when you clench your back teeth together) and massage them in a slow, circular motion. Move your fingertips back slightly to another tense spot of the jaw and again massage in a slow, circular motion, taking long, deep breaths; cover an area the size of a nickel.

3. With the heels of your hands, slowly rub the skin up and down the sides of your face from your jaws to your temples; do this several times as you take long, deep breaths.

4. Again massage the sides of your face, this time in a circular motion with your fingertips, using firm pressure on the jaw muscles; the temples also benefit from being massaged in this way.

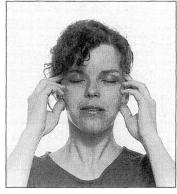

This exercise is good for sinusitis, headaches, the brain, nervous system, and jaw problems.

28
KNEE PAIN

The knee joints absorb much of the body's weight when we stand or move. People who engage in running sports, skiing, or skating often complain of knee pain, as do people who are overweight. Whether the pain is due to acute strain or a chronic muscular problem, acupressure helps relieve pain, reduces swelling, and increases blood circulation to the knee area.

To relieve pain in an affected knee and to prevent injuries to healthy knees, spend ten minutes three times a day for a few weeks thoroughly massaging the painful knee using the following methods and points: First, apply hot compresses with a thick, heavy towel that has been soaked in hot water or use a heating pad until the heat penetrates deep into the knee joint. Once the joint is warmed up, practice the following knee pain "Potent Point Exercises." Try to stay off your legs during this time (for example, avoid stairs as much as possible) to give your knee the rest necessary to enable it to heal.

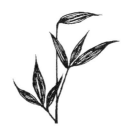

Potent Points for Relieving Knee Pain

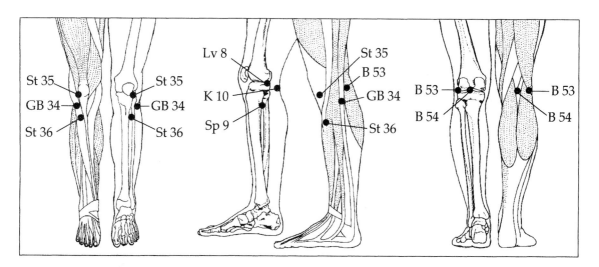

Commanding Middle (B 54)

Location: In the center of the back of the knee in the crease of the knee joint.

Benefits: Relieves knee pain, stiffness, arthritis, back pain, and sciatica.

Crooked Spring (Lv 8)

Location: On the inside of the knee, where the crease ends when the knee is bent.

Benefits: Relieves knee pain, fibroids, and swelling in the knee.

Nourishing Valley (K 10)

Location: On the inner edge of the knee crease, in the hollow between two tendons.

Benefits: Knee pain, genital disorders, and abdominal pain.

Shady Side of the Mountain (Sp 9)

Location: On the inside of the leg, just below the bulge that is down from the inside of the knee and under the head of the shinbone.

Benefits: Relieves knee problems, swelling, leg tensions, varicose veins, edema, water retention, and cramps.

Sunny Side of the Mountain (GB 34)

Location: On the outside of the lower leg, below and in front of the head of the shinbone.

Benefits: Relieves excessive knee pain, muscular tension, aches, and muscle strains.

Commanding Activity (B 53)

Location: On the outside of the knee, where the crease ends when the knee is bent.

Benefits: Relieves knee pain and stiffness.

Calf's Nose (St 35)

Location: Just below the kneecap in the outer indentation.

Benefits: Relieves knee pain, knee stiffness, rheumatism of the feet, and edema.

Three Mile Point (St 36)

Location: Four finger widths below the kneecap, one finger outside of the shinbone.

Benefits: Strengthens the whole body, tones the muscles, and relieves knee pain.

■ *You do not have to use all of these points. Using just one or two of them can be effective.*

Potent Point Exercises

Sit comfortably on a rug or mat, up against a wall to support your back. Extend your legs in front of you. Breathe deeply as you stimulate each of the following acupressure points.

Step 1

Use a tennis ball to press B 54: Place the tennis ball in the middle of the crease behind the affected knee. If you place the tennis ball on a thick pillow it will prevent the ball from slipping and support your knee more comfortably. Keep the ball in this position while completing the rest of the steps.

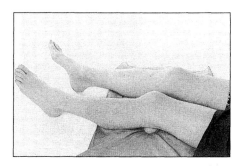

Step 2

Rub Lv 8, Sp 9, K 10, B 53, and GB 34: Place the palms of your hands on both sides of your knee, covering these points. Briskly rub both sides for one minute to create a warming friction.

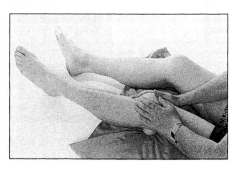

Step 3

Press around the kneecap and on St 35: Use the thumbs and index fingers of both hands to press around the sides of your kneecap,

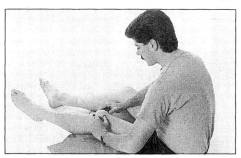

directing your pressure underneath the knee bone. This stimulates St 35 as well as other special knee points. Lean your weight forward to apply the pressure for ten seconds. Then release the pressure, rotate your fingertips one quarter of an inch and gradually reapply the pressure underneath your kneecap. Repeat this several times to thoroughly press around the kneecap for two minutes.

If you have pain when you attempt to rotate your kneecap, skip this step and proceed to the next exercise.

Step 4

Rotate the kneecap: Grasp your kneecap in the palm of your hand, then slowly rotate in one direction ten times, then in the opposite direction ten times, as you breathe deeply.

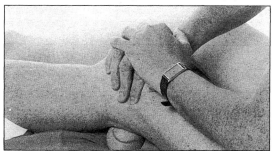

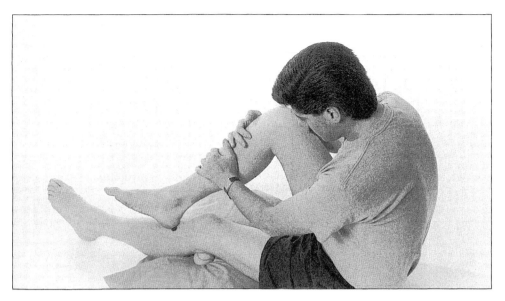

Step 5

Briskly rub St 36: Place your opposite heel on St 36, three inches below your kneecap on the outside of your leg. Briskly rub your heel over this point, creating heat from the friction, for thirty seconds.

Step 6

Leg and knee stretch: Gradually lean forward, flexing your toes toward you and pushing your heel away from you as you slowly count to five, then take a deep breath and let your leg relax. Repeat this stretch two more times.

Step 7
Repeat step 2.

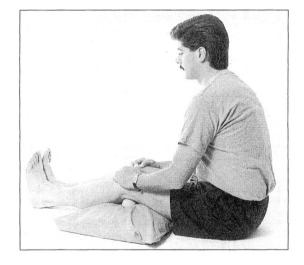

Step 8

Switch legs: Repeat steps 1 through 7 on your other leg. Spend twice as much time on the leg and knee that are giving you the most trouble.

Additional Points for Relieving Knee Pain

For illustrations of other related points for relieving knee pain, see chapter 5, "Ankle and Foot Problems"; chapter 9, "Backache and Sciatica"; and chapter 35, "Pain."

29

LABOR, DELIVERY, AND NURSING

*J*ean, one of my main instructors at the Acupressure Institute, was working with a pregnant woman whose delivery was three weeks late. The mother had intermittent contractions: they would start up but then taper off. After Jean worked with the woman for thirty minutes, holding the trigger points on her hands and ankles, the contractions became more regular, and the mother actually felt the baby respond to the finger pressure; there was a tremendous increase in the baby's movements. Jean also showed the mother many self-acupressure points and techniques that gave her greater confidence during the labor and relief from the pain and exhaustion.

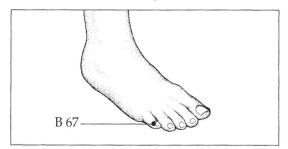

B 67

When B 67 on the mother's little toe was stimulated in the hospital, she felt the baby drop into position. The acupressure helped the mother relax, and she was able to have more control of her pain during the birth.

Self-acupressure can greatly ease the stress and pain of childbirth without causing any of the side effects of drugs. Tension and fatigue tend to increase labor pain — the more you resist the pain, the stronger it gets — so relaxation is key to easing labor. Acupressure used with deep breathing releases muscle tension and helps you relax.

By pressing the restorative points illustrated in this chapter, you can boost your overall system during pregnancy, as well as prepare for the delivery. There are also several postpartum recovery points that relieve muscle soreness, stimulate lactation, and restore vitality after childbirth.

Participating in caring for yourself during labor builds the self-confidence you need to deal with the anxiety and fear that often arise. Perhaps the most exciting aspect of using acupressure during labor and delivery, however, is the deeper connection you feel not only to your own body, but also with your new baby.

Caution: You must call your doctor, midwife, and/or care coordinator when labor begins and be prepared to get to the hospital.

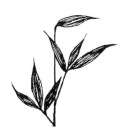

Potent Points for Relieving Labor Pain

Shoulder Well (GB 21)

Caution: Do not apply harsh or sudden pressure on this point. Instead, gradually apply pressure on pregnant women.

Location: On the top of the shoulder, directly on the muscle, one to two inches out from the side of the lower neck.

Benefits: Assists childbirth and relieves pain, nervousness, irritability, fatigue, shoulder tension, poor circulation, cold hands and feet.

Sacral Points (B 27-B 34)

The acupressure points at the sacrum (the large bony area at the base of the spine) help relieve menstrual cramps, and lower-back and labor pain. Steady, firm pressure on these sacral points — by lying on your back with your hands, one on top of the other, under the base of the spine — helps relax the uterus and the pelvic area to relieve pain during labor.

Joining the Valley (Hoku) (LI 4)

Location: In the webbing between the thumb and index finger at the highest spot of the muscle when the thumb and index finger are brought close together.

Benefits: Relieves labor pain, constipation, headaches, toothaches, shoulder pain, and arthritis.

Bigger Stream (K 3)

Caution: Do not stimulate this point strongly after the third month of pregnancy.

Location: Midway between the inner protrusions of the anklebone and the Achilles tendon in the back of the ankle.

Benefits: Relieves labor pain, swollen feet, fatigue, ankle pain, and back pain.

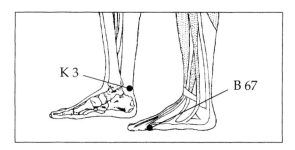

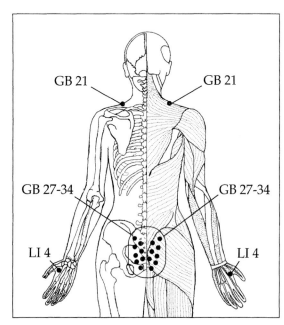

■ *You do not have to use all of these points. Using just one or two of them can be effective.*

Reaching Inside (B 67)

Location: On the outside of the little toe, at the base of the toenail.

Benefits: Used for difficult labor, malposition of the fetus,[40] nasal obstruction, and itchy skin.

---

[40] To prevent a breech birth, heat can be used on this trigger point to stimulate the fetus to change its position in the womb during the last trimester of the pregnancy. Consult with your physician and then with an acupressurist or acupuncturist for further details.

Potent Point Exercises for Labor Pain

The following routine can be practiced while sitting comfortably or lying down. It may be easier to stimulate the points on your feet in a sitting position. Concentrate on taking long, slow, deep breaths as you hold the following points on your body. Each of these acupressure techniques can be done by your partner, a friend, or your labor coach. The following instructions can be practiced in full as a complete routine or in part, combining just a couple of the steps.

Step 1

Gradually press GB 21: Curve your fingers, placing your fingertips directly on the muscle on the top of your shoulders close to your neck. Breathe deeply as you gradually press into any shoulder tension at this spot for one minute.

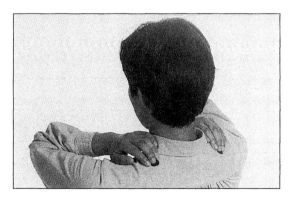

Step 2

Press or rub B 27-B 34: Press these points for delivery. Use the backs of your hands to briskly rub the base of your spine, creating warmth from the friction. If you can comfortably lie down on your back for a couple of minutes, place your hands one on top of the other, underneath the base of your spine. Bend your knees with your feet flat on

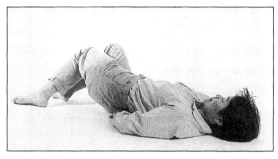

the bed. Breathe deeply as you slowly rock your pelvis left and right to stimulate these sacral points. This relaxes your pelvic region and encourages your cervix to dilate.

Step 3

Firmly press LI 4: Place your right thumb on the back of your left hand in the webbing between the thumb and index finger, with your fingertips on the palm directly behind your thumb. Squeeze the thumb and index finger of your right hand together to firmly press into the webbing. Angle the pressure underneath the bone that connects with the index finger. To expedite labor, stimulate the point by rubbing it; to relieve labor pain, grip the webbing firmer and hold it longer. Hold the point for one minute as you breathe deeply into your belly. Then switch sides to work on your other hand.

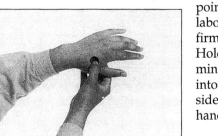

Labor Pain Relief Points: Show your labor coach or friend the following potent points.

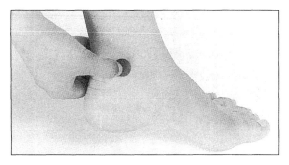

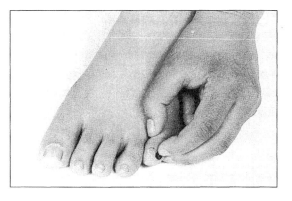

Firmly press K 3: Bend your leg, placing your thumb between your inner anklebone and the Achilles tendon; press this point to ease labor pains. Hold one side at a time for a minute each, or reposition your body to hold both points simultaneously.

Stimulate B 67: Use the nail of your index finger to gently scratch B 67 on the outside of the nail of the little toe. Stimulate each side for thirty seconds.

Postpartum Recovery Potent Points

Sea of Energy (CV 6)

Location: Two finger widths below the belly button.

Benefits: Relieves weak abdominal muscles, lower-back pain, kidney pain, constipation, gas, uroreproductive problems, irregular vaginal discharge, general weakness, and insomnia.

Inner Gate (P 6)

Location: In the middle of the inner side of the forearm, two and one-half finger widths from the wrist crease.

Benefits: Relieves postpartum discomfort, insomnia, anxiety, palpitations, wrist pain, nausea, and indigestion.

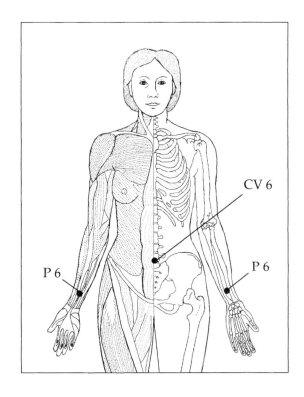

Sea of Vitality (B 23 and B 47)

Caution: Do not press on disintegrating discs or fractured or broken bones. If you have a weak back, a few minutes of stationary, light touching instead of pressure can be very healing. See your doctor first if you have any questions or need medical advice.

Location: On the lower back (between the second and third lumbar vertebrae), two and four finger widths away from the spine at waist level.

Benefits: Relieves postpartum discomfort, lower-back aches, fatigue, sexual-reproductive problems, impotency, irregular vaginal discharge, and urinary problems.

Womb and Vitals (B 48)

Location: One to two finger widths outside the large bony area at the base of the spine (sacrum) and midway between the top of the hipbone (iliac crest) and the base of the buttock.

Benefits: Relieves pelvic tension, bladder weakness, constipation, hemorrhoids, urinary problems, sciatica, lower backaches, hip pain, and frustration.

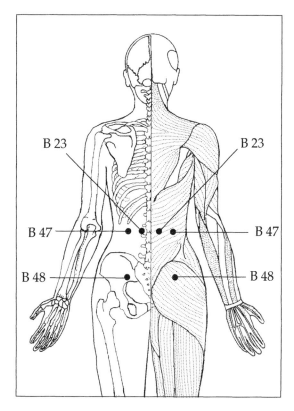

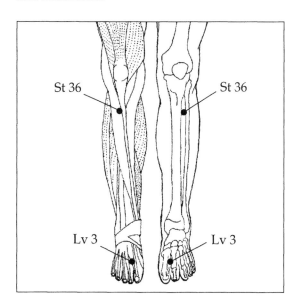

Three Mile Point (St 36)

Location: Four finger widths below the kneecap, one finger width outside of the shinbone. If you are on the correct spot, a muscle should flex as you move your foot up and down.

Benefits: Used for postpartum recovery, strengthens and tones the muscles, aids digestion, and relieves stomach disorders and fatigue.

Bigger Rushing (Lv 3)

Location: On the top of the foot, in the valley between the big toe and the second toe.

Benefits: Relieves continuous sweating that can occur after childbirth, cramps, headaches, and eye fatigue.

■ *You do not have to use all of these points. Using just one or two of them whenever you have a free hand can be effective.*

Potent Point Exercises for Postpartum Recovery

Lie down comfortably on your back or in the fetal position and take long, deep breaths as you hold the following points.

Step 1

Press B 23 and B 47: Make fists and place them under your lower back. Use your knuckles to press the thick, ropy muscles of your lower back at the level of your waist. This pressure stimulates both the inner lower back point B 23 and the outer point B 47 at the same time. Take long, slow, deep breaths into your abdomen for two minutes.

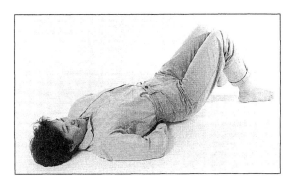

Step 2

Press B 48: Move your fists lower, underneath your buttocks, on either side of the base of your spine. As your knuckles press B 48, take long, deep breaths and let your head gently roll from side to side for one minute.

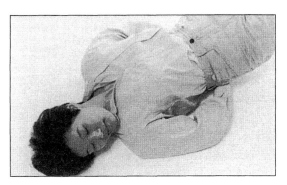

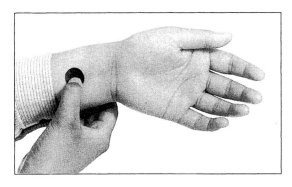

Step 3

Firmly press P 6: Place your right thumb on the inside of your wrist, two and one-half finger widths from the crease. Pressing firmly for thirty seconds. Then switch sides to press your other wrist.

Step 4

Firmly press CV 6: Place all of your fingertips into your lower abdominal area, between your belly button and pubic bone. Close your eyes and breathe deeply into this point for two minutes. Let yourself relax deeply after pressing CV 6; it's one of the most powerful postpartum recovery points. A short nap after pressing this point can be especially healing.

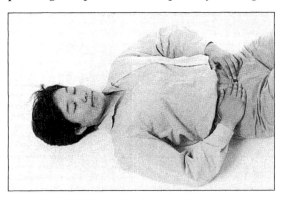

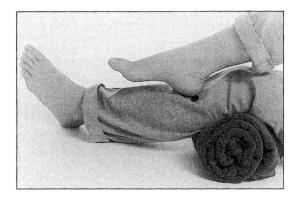

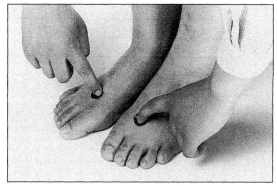

Step 5

Press St 36: Place your right heel on the left leg just outside and slightly below the kneecap. Press St 36 with your heel. After thirty seconds, do the same on your other leg. Take a minute to hold this potent point gently several times a day to strengthen your entire body after childbirth.

Step 6

Stimulate Lv 3: Slowly sit up, placing your fingertips or your opposite heel on the top of the foot in the valley between the bones that connect with the large and second toes. Firmly rub into the groove to stimulate Lv 3 on both sides for thirty seconds. Then lie down, close your eyes, and deeply relax.

Potent Points for Nursing

Letting Go (Lu 1)

Location: On the outer part of the chest, three finger widths below the collarbone. If you're on the right spot, you should feel the muscle bulge when you pull your arm into your body and tense the arm.

Benefits: Relieves breathing difficulties, fatigue, confusion, chest tension and congestion, emotional repression, coughing, and asthma.

Breast Window (St 16)

Location: Directly above the breast tissue in line with the nipples, between the third and fourth ribs.

Benefits: Relieves breast pains, lactation problems, heartburn, insomnia, depression, and chest congestion.

Heavenly Pond (P 1)

Location: One thumb width outside the nipple.

Benefits: Breast and chest pain, lymph glands, and insufficient milk during nursing.

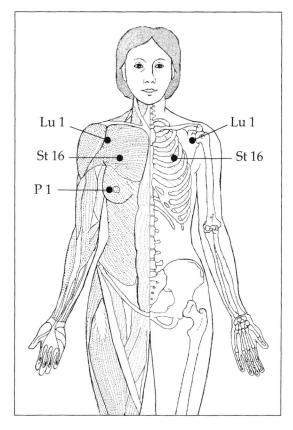

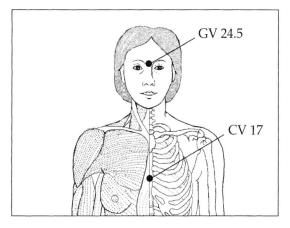

■ *You do not have to use all of these points. Using just one or two of them whenever you have a free hand can be effective.*

Third Eye Point (GV 24.5)

Location: Directly between the eyebrows, in the indentation where the bridge of the nose meets the forehead.

Benefits: Used for breastfeeding difficulties, glandular imbalances; also relieves hay fever, headaches, indigestion, ulcer pain, and eyestrain.

Sea of Tranquility (CV 17)

Location: On the center of the breastbone three thumb widths up from the base of the bone.

Benefits: Relieves nervousness, chest congestion, insomnia, anguish, depression, hysteria, and other emotional imbalances.

Potent Point Exercises

The following acupressure routine can be practiced either sitting or lying down comfortably.

Step 1

Press Lu 1: Curve your fingers and place your right fingertips on the upper, outer portion of the left side of your chest, and your left fingertips on the right side of your chest.

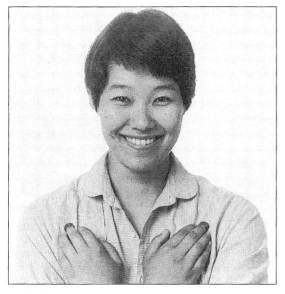

Make firm contact with the muscles located four finger widths up and one finger width inward from your armpit crease as you breathe deeply, holding for one minute with your eyes closed.

Step 2

Lightly press St 16: Place your middle fingertips just above the breast on the nipple line to feel for a sore, tender spot. Hold this point for one minute as you breathe deeply.

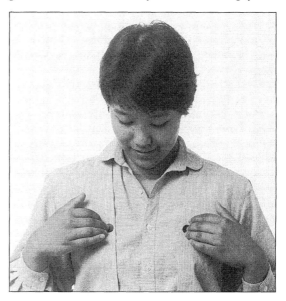

Step 3

Lightly press P 1: Place your fingertips beside your nipple to lightly hold P 1 for one minute on both sides. Please note that this step is not shown here. For an illustration of P 1 please refer to the previous page.

Step 4

Hold GV 24.5 along with CV 17: Place the third fingertip of your right hand lightly on the Third Eye Point, between your eyebrows. Use your left fingertips to hold CV 17, at the center of your breastbone. Close your eyes and take long, slow, deep breaths for one to two minutes to calm, nourish, and relax yourself and bask in your own healing.

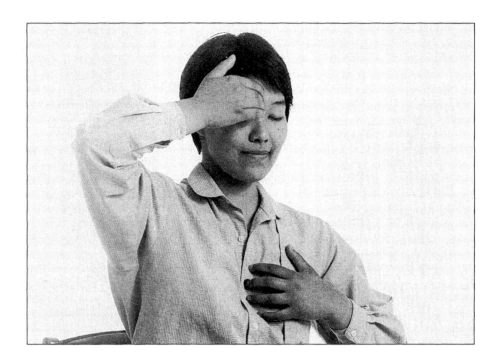

Additional Points for Labor, Delivery, and Nursing

For illustrations of other related points for relieving labor and delivery pain, see chapter 36, "Pregnancy and Infertility."

30
MEMORY AND CONCENTRATION

*Y*ou can enhance your powers of concentration by using a combination of acupressure and proper diet. When you are under a great deal of stress or when your gastrointestinal system is weak or congested, thinking clearly is difficult. Similarly, if you eat a hearty meal and then try to study or read a technical article, you'll find it hard to concentrate. Chronic tension in the shoulder and neck, for instance, can also contribute to memory troubles by inhibiting the circulation of blood to the brain. As this tension accumulates over the years, it can cause chronic fatigue and poor concentration. Anyone who studies for hours at a time or does close, concentrated detail work should use the points in this chapter, as well as the self-acupressure techniques illustrated in chapter 37, Shoulder Tension.

Memory and power of concentration do not have to get worse with age. You can retard the aging process to a large degree by working on yourself with acupressure and by eating the right foods. You should also consult a physician if you have chronically poor memory to make sure that an underlying condition such as heart disease or high blood pressure is not affecting your mental functions. Medications of many sorts also have deleterious effects on short-term memory.

Diet

If you have difficulty concentrating or want to improve your memory, you should stop eating foods that are high in sugar. Sugar tends to be addicting and keeps people from eating other nutritious foods. Eating a lot of sugar also strains the pancreas, which according to traditional Chinese medicine is damaging to your memory as well as your mental

and emotional stability.

Poor memory and concentration also can be the result of a low blood sugar level. Shortly after eating sugar, your blood sugar level rises, producing a burst of energy. To balance this sharp increase, however, the pancreas overproduces insulin; too much insulin drastically lowers the blood sugar level, causing fatigue and impairing memory and the ability to concentrate. To stabilize your blood sugar levels, try eating more complex carbohydrates such as fresh vegetables and whole grains. Complex carbohydrates are broken down into sugar in the bloodstream at a slower rate, which keeps the blood sugar level steady. Miso soup, gota kola herbal tea, fresh wheat grass juice, and sprouts (all available in health food stores) are also excellent foods for balancing blood sugar levels and for benefiting the memory.

Acupressure for Mental Clarity

The acupressure point formula in this chapter improves alertness and memory by increasing blood circulation to the brain. Finger pressure on these points for up to two minutes is good for relieving mental fatigue and headaches, and for improving memory. These points can instantly refresh you and clear your mind. A calm, relaxed state of mind encourages greater productivity and a positive outlook on life. You can also teach your child these points.

Stimulate each of the following acupressure points on both sides of the body in the order given for a minute or two. Practice this routine sitting comfortably or lying down, several times a week (daily is best), to enhance your memory and increase your powers of concentration.

Potent Points for Improving Memory and Concentration

One Hundred Meeting Point (GV 20)

Location: On the crown of the head in between the cranial bones. To find the point, follow the line from the back of both ears to the top of the head. Feel for a slight hollow toward the back of the top of the head.

Benefits: Good for mental concentration and improving memory; relieves headaches.

Sun Point (EX 2)

Location: In the depression of the temples, one-half inch to the outside of the eyebrows.

Benefits: Improves memory and concentration; relieves mental stress, headaches, and dizziness.

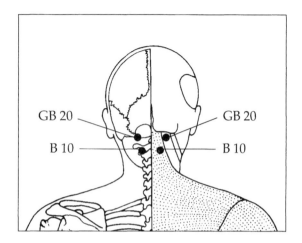

Heavenly Pillar (B 10)

Location: One-half inch below the base of the skull on the ropy muscles one-half inch outward from the spine.

Benefits: Relieves stress, burnout, overexertion, heaviness in the head, and unclear thinking. This point will help relax your neck allowing greater circulation into your brain.

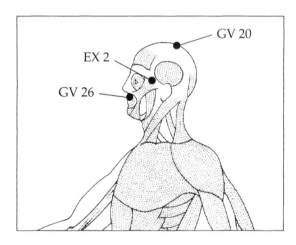

Middle of a Person (GV 26)

Location: Two-thirds of the way up from the upper lip to the nose.

Benefits: Improves memory and concentration, and relieves cramps, fainting, and dizziness. The effectiveness of this point often increases by pressing it firmly each day over a period of several weeks.

Gates of Consciousness (GB 20)

Location: Below the base of the skull, in the hollows on both sides about two to three inches apart depending on the size of the head.

Benefits: Remedies headaches, poor memory, and relieves arthritic pain that inhibits the ability to concentrate, regardless of the pain's location.

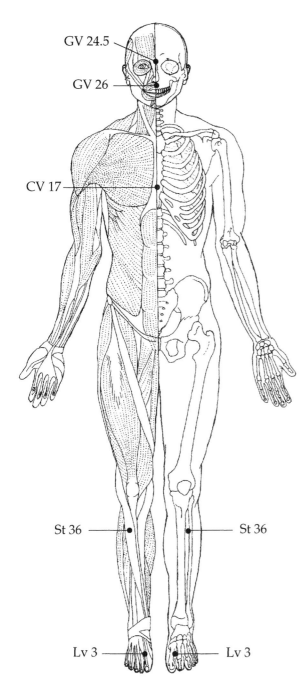

GV 24.5

GV 26

CV 17

St 36 — St 36

Lv 3 — Lv 3

Third Eye Point (GV 24.5)

Location: Directly between the eyebrows, in the indentation where the bridge of the nose meets the forehead.

Benefits: Good for improving concentration and memory; clears the mind and uplifts the spirit.

Sea of Tranquility (CV 17)

Location: On the center of the breastbone three thumb widths up from the base of the bone.

Benefits: Aids concentration; relieves nervousness, chest congestion, insomnia, depression, anxiety, and other emotional imbalances that inhibit concentration and clear thinking.

Three Mile Point (St 36)

Location: Four finger widths below the kneecap, one finger width outside of the shinbone. If you are on the correct spot, a muscle should flex as you move your foot up and down.

Benefits: Strengthens the mind and body as well as aiding mental clarity.

Bigger Rushing (Lv 3)

Location: On the top of the foot, in the valley between the big toe and the second toe.

Benefits: Relieves poor memory, headaches, fatigue, and poor concentration.

■ *You do not have to use all of these points. Using just one or two of them whenever you have a free hand can be effective.*

Potent Point Exercises

Practice the following routine sitting comfortably or lying down. Stimulate these potent points twice a day for best results.

Step 1

Hold GV 20 along with GV 26: Place the fingertips of your left hand in the indentation in the center of the top of your head toward the back. Use your right index finger to press

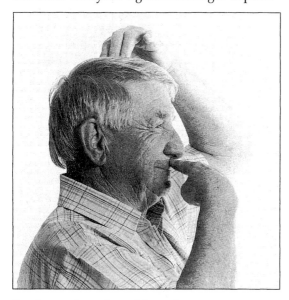

firmly on the point midway between your upper lip and your nose, angling pressure into the upper gum. Breathe deeply as you hold this potent point combination for one minute.

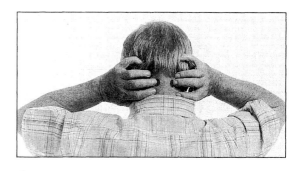

Step 2

Firmly press B 10: Use all of your fingertips to press firmly into the ropy muscles on the back of your neck. Hold this point for one minute as you breathe deeply.

Step 3

Press GB 20: Place your thumbs underneath the base of your skull in the indentations that lie about two and one-half to three inches apart. Slowly tilt your head back as you

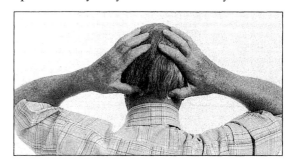

gradually press up and under the skull. Close your eyes and breathe deeply as you firmly press into these points for two minutes. Finish by holding these points lightly to feel for a pulsation. The pulse indicates that there is greater circulation traveling through your brain, which can improve your memory and concentration. If you continue to hold these points long enough, the pulses on both sides will synchronize and balance both hemispheres of the brain. Then very slowly release the pressure.

Step 4

Palm EX 2: Position the heel of your hands on your temples in the indentations just outside your eyebrows. If you're sitting near a desk or table, lean your elbows on it while you apply pressure in the temples with the heel of your hands. After a minute of firm pressure in the temples, begin to rhythmically clench your back molars together as if you are chewing gum. Each time you clench your teeth together, you should feel a muscle pop out in your temples. Close your eyes and continue to press your temples firmly as you chew and breathe deeply for at least one minute. This strongly stimulates this point and strengthens your memory and concentration.

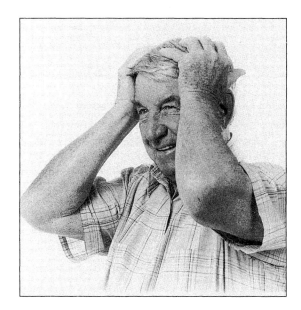

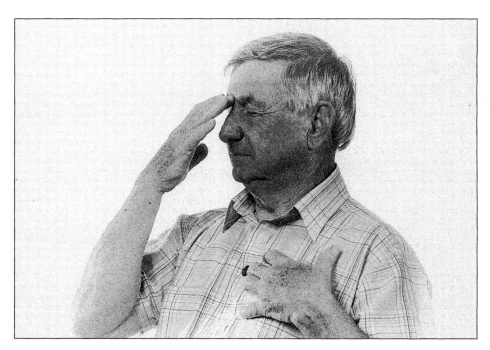

Step 5

Hold GV 24.5 along with CV 17.
Place your right middle fingertip lightly between your eyebrows in the indentation where the bridge of the nose meets the forehead. Use your left fingertips to press the indentations on the center of your breastbone. Close your eyes, raising your eyes upward as you imagine you are breathing into and out of the Third Eye Point for one or two minutes.

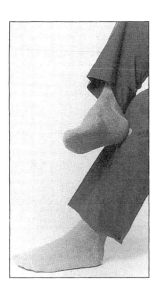

Step 6

Briskly rub St 36: Place your right heel on the outside of your left leg just below the knee. Rub up and down just outside of the shinbone to create heat from the friction for thirty seconds. Then switch sides and rub St 36 on your right leg for thirty seconds.

Step 7

Press or rub Lv 3: Place your right heel on the top of your left foot in the groove between the bones that connect with your big and second

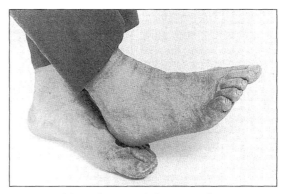

toes. Briskly rub up and down in this groove. Then switch sides to press the point on your right foot for another thirty seconds.

Additional Points for Improving Memory and Concentration

For illustrations of other related points for improving memory and concentration, see chapter 12, "Constipation"; chapter 18, "Fainting"; and chapter 20, "Headaches and Migraines."

31

MENSTRUAL TENSION, CRAMPS, AND PMS

*W*omen often experience lower-back aches, bloating, breast tenderness, and abdominal cramping before or during menstruation. The special acupressure points in this chapter not only release tension in these areas but also help reduce menstrual discomfort and bloating, stabilize your emotions, and help you gain more control over your life.

Menstrual problems can be caused by pelvic tension; uterine inflammation and swelling; constipation; a contracted cervix; and hormonal imbalances of the thyroid, parathyroid, or ovaries. You should always consult your physician to determine what might be causing your problems. Daily acupressure over a period of time stimulates the endocrine system to regulate these hormones naturally. This kind of natural treatment method takes longer to produce results but has none of the side effects of drugs, so discuss this alternative with your physician.

Pelvic tension, another common cause of PMS and menstrual cramps, directly affects the reproductive and digestive organs. When the muscles of the pelvic area contract, the colon can become blocked, and the circulation of both blood and nerve signals to the genitals is decreased, affecting menstrual flow. The acupressure points in the groin and at the base of the spine release pelvic tension by increasing the circulation throughout the reproductive system.

Diet

Calcium is one of the most important minerals for preventing menstrual cramps. It enables the nerves and muscles to relax. Calcium levels drop substantially during the week before menstruation, causing premenstrual tension, bloating, and headaches.

Many foods supply the body with calcium and can thus help prevent cramps if eaten the week before menstruation. Fresh leafy green vegetables such as lettuce, spinach, kale, parsley (which can be steeped for tea), collards, and turnip greens are high in calcium. Magnesium is also important, because it facilitates the body's absorption of calcium. Sea vegetables, seeds, and nuts contain high amounts of both these minerals.

Tips for Relieving Menstrual Discomforts

- **Camomile tea** is good for relieving PMS and menstrual cramps; it soothes, calms, and relaxes the system.

- **Fresh ginger root tea** is also an excellent remedy for menstrual cramps. Ginger root is available in the produce department of most markets. Slice a handful and simmer it in water for fifteen minutes. Add a little honey and milk to taste. Enjoy a cup or two.

- **Apply a hot water bottle**, heating pad, or hot towel to the small of the back. Then loosely cover the body with a blanket.

- **Apply a light mustard plaster** to the abdomen. Mix one part ground mustard seed with five parts whole wheat flour. Mix with warm water to make a paste thick enough to spread on a piece of cheesecloth. Then place the cheesecloth over the lower abdomen. Leave on until it fully warms the abdomen. After removing the mustard plaster, lie down and cover yourself.

- **Hot or cold applications** can also ease menstrual tension. Heat from a sauna or bath increases menstrual flow; cold decreases it.

Potent Points for Relieving PMS

Rushing Door (Sp 12)
Mansion Cottage (Sp 13)

These two points are very important for releasing menstrual discomforts

Location: In the pelvic area, in the middle of the crease where the leg joins the trunk of the body.

Benefits: Relieves menstrual cramps and abdominal discomfort.

Sacral Points (B 27-B 34)

The acupressure points on the sacrum (at the base of the spine directly above the tail bone) help relieve menstrual cramps and lower-back pain. Two minutes of steady, firm pressure on these sacral points — by lying down on your back with your hands, one on top of the other, under the base of the spine — helps relax the uterus and relieve menstrual cramps.

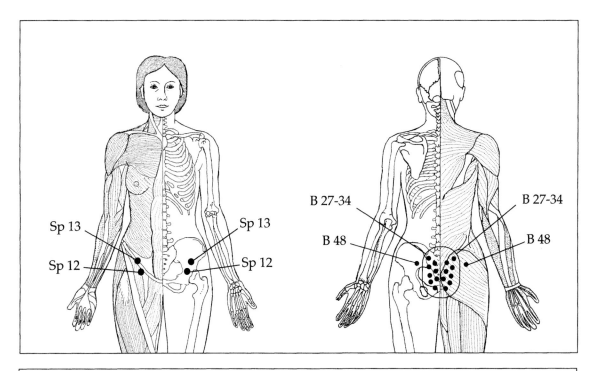

Point Number	Benefits and Uses
B 27, B 28	Relieves hip pain, menstrual cramps, retention of urine, and reproductive problems.
B 29, B 30	Relieves lower-back pain, sciatica, and sacral pain due to menstruation.
B 31, B 32	Relieves PMS and menstrual tension.
B 33, B 34	Lumbago, genital pain, impotency, and sterility.

Sea of Energy (CV 6)

Location: Two finger widths below the belly button.

Benefits: Relieves PMS, menstrual cramps, uroreproductive problems, irregular vaginal discharge, irregular periods, and constipation that increases menstrual pain.

Gate Origin (CV 4)

Location: Four finger widths below the belly button.

Benefits: Relieves menstrual cramps, uroreproductive problems, irregular vaginal discharge, irregular menstrual periods, and incontinence.

Womb and Vitals (B 48)

Location: One to two finger widths outside the sacrum (the large bony area at the base of the spine) and midway between the top of the hipbone (iliac crest) and the base of the buttocks.

Benefits: Relieves pelvic tension, PMS, menstrual cramps, and urinary problems.

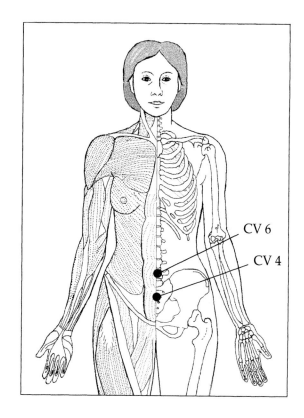

CV 6
CV 4

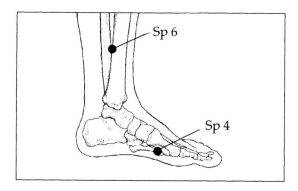

Sp 6

Sp 4

■ *You do not have to use all of these points. Using just one or two of them can be quite effective whenever you feel PMS or cramps developing.*

Three Yin Crossing (Sp 6)

Caution: Do not stimulate this point during the eighth and ninth months of pregnancy.

Location: Four finger widths above the inner anklebone close to the back of the shinbone.

Benefits: Relieves water retention, menstrual cramps, irregular vaginal discharge, and genital pain.

Grandfather Grandson (Sp 4)

Location: In the upper arch of the foot, one thumb width from the ball of the foot.

Benefits: Relieves PMS, bloating, and menstrual and abdominal cramps.

169

Potent Point Exercises

Practice the following self-care techniques in a quiet, comfortable, private room. For best results, practice two or three times a day for the week before your period and once a day throughout the rest of the month. This routine uses three positions: first lie on your stomach to work on your groin; second, lie on your back to work on your buttocks and the base of your spine; and third, sit up to press two important points on the insides of your legs to rebalance the female reproductive system.

Step 1

Press Sp 12 and Sp 13: Lie flat on your stomach, and place your arms underneath your body with your fists underneath your groin, closed palms facing up. Put your forehead or chin on the floor, whichever is most comfortable. Bring your feet together. Inhale, and raise your feet up with your thighs off the ground. Begin long, deep breathing into your belly with your legs up for thirty seconds. Then slowly come down, bringing your hands by your sides, turning your head on its side and adjust your body comfortably to completely relax for at least two minutes.

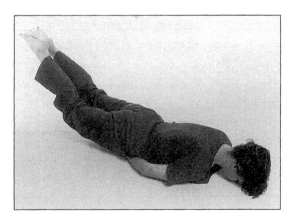

Slowly roll over onto your back.

Step 2

Press B 48 and B 27-B 34: Lie on your back with your legs bent, feet flat on the floor. Place your hands flat on the floor, palms facing down, underneath your buttocks beside the base of your spine (sacrum). Close your eyes and take long, deep breaths as your knees sway from side to side for one minute.

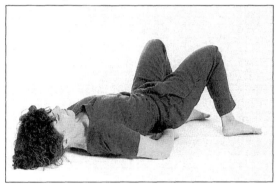

Reposition your hands underneath your buttocks both for comfort and to press different parts of the buttock muscles. Then move your hands closer inward, underneath the base of the spine. If you find a particularly tender spot, hold the area for one minute and breathe deeply.

Also try this exercise with your knees pulled closer to your abdomen and your feet off the floor. Keep your hands underneath your buttocks as you rock your knees from side to side. After another minute, extend your legs outward, placing your hands on your belly and breathe deeply. Let yourself completely relax for a couple of minutes with your eyes closed.

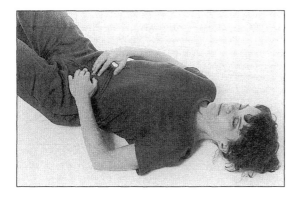

Step 3

Gradually press CV 4 and CV 6: Place the fingertips of your left hand in the center of your abdomen just above your pubic bone (CV 4). Position your right fingertips directly above this, in the center between your belly button and pubic bone (CV 6). Breathe deeply into your belly as you gradually press one to two inches deep inside the abdomen and hold for two minutes. Then completely relax on your back with your eyes closed for as long as you like.

Roll onto your side and slowly come up to a comfortable sitting position.

Step 4

Gently press Sp 6: Place both of your thumbs on the inside of your ankles, four finger widths above the protrusion of the inner

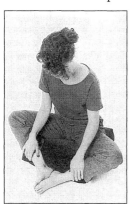

anklebone. Gently rub your thumbs on the inner border of the shinbone, feeling for a slight indentation to gently press into. If you have PMS or menstrual cramps, this point will probably be very tender. Hold for one minute as you breathe deeply.

Step 5

Firmly press Sp 4: Place your thumbs on the arches of your feet, with your right hand on your right foot, and your left hand on your left foot. With your thumbs on the arch of each foot, wiggle your toes back and forth to feel a muscle pop out. Firmly press that muscle for one minute.

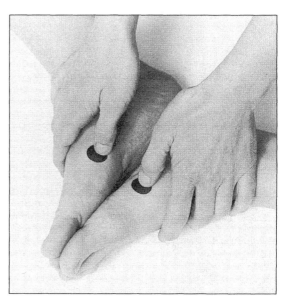

For best results, practice this routine two or three times a day for the week before your period, and once a day throughout the rest of the month.

Additional Points for Relieving Menstrual Cramps and PMS

For illustrations of related points for relieving menstrual tension and PMS, see chapter 9, "Backache and Sciatica"; chapter 13, "Cramps and Spasms"; and chapter 35, "Pain."

32

MOTION SICKNESS, MORNING SICKNESS, AND NAUSEA

*I*n classes and lectures, I have shown hundreds of people how they can use self-acupressure to relieve nausea, motion sickness, air sickness, and even seasickness. Press both sides of the trigger point P 6 (described in the middle of the next page); it works in just a few minutes. My sister used this point during her pregnancy to relieve her morning sickness.

Nausea can be caused by nervousness, indigestion, abdominal imbalances, and ingestion of chemicals or poisons, including certain drugs and alcohol. Many medical disorders such as stomach cancer, gastritis, stomach ulcers, meningitis, and diabetes — to name just a few — can also produce nausea,

so if your nausea is severe or persistent, call your doctor.

Acupressure can relieve nausea, especially in cases where it is caused or worsened by physical or emotional distress. When tension accumulates in the stomach, it inhibits proper abdominal circulation, puts stress on the digestive tract, and can make you feel sick. Gentle acupressure applied locally at the base of the rib cage, along with two trigger points on the inside of the wrist, relieve nausea. You can teach these points to your child for motion sickness or stomach flu, and these same points are effective for relieving morning sickness.

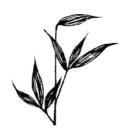

Potent Points for Relieving Motion Sickness, Morning Sickness, and Nausea

Heavenly Appearance (SI 17)

Location: In the indentation between the earlobe and the tip of the jawbone.

Benefits: Relieves nausea, ear pain, facial paralysis or spasms, jaw pain, itching in the ears, and swollen throat.

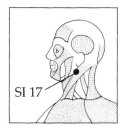

Intermediary (P 5)

Location: Four finger widths above the center of the inner wrist crease, between the tendons.

Benefits: Relieves upset stomach, nausea, and vomiting.

Inner Gate (P 6)

Location: In the middle of the inner side of the forearm two and one-half finger widths above the wrist crease.

Benefits: Relieves nausea, indigestion, stomachaches, and wrist pain.

Abdominal Sorrow (Sp 16)

Location: Below the edge of the rib cage (at the junction of the ninth rib cartilage to the eighth rib) in line with the earlobe.

Benefits: Relieves indigestion, appetite imbalances, abdominal cramps, and hiccups.

Three Mile Point (St 36)

Location: Four finger widths below the kneecap, one finger width outside of the shinbone. A muscle should flex as you move your foot up and down.

Benefits: Aids digestion and relieves nausea, stomach disorders, and fatigue.

Bigger Rushing (Lv 3)

Location: On the top of the foot, in the valley between the big toe and the second toe.

Benefits: Relieves nausea and cramps.

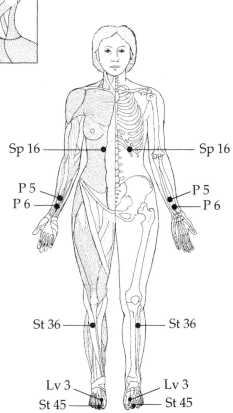

Severe Mouth (St 45)

Location: On the outside of the base of the nail of the second toe.

Benefits: Relieves nausea, indigestion, food poisoning, toothaches, and abdominal pain.

■ *You do not have to use all of these points. Using just one or two of them whenever you have a free hand can be effective.*

Potent Point Exercises

The following routine can be done anywhere, at any time, in a comfortable sitting position.

Step 1

Lightly press SI 17: Place your middle and index fingertips just below your earlobe.

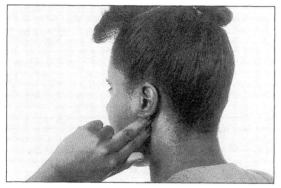

Gradually apply a light pressure as you breathe deeply for one minute. This point is usually ultrasensitive to finger pressure. Be careful; apply your finger pressure slowly and gently.

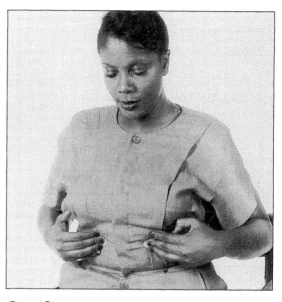

Step 3

Hold Sp 16: Curve your fingers and place them on the base of your rib cage directly below your nipple. Hold these points firmly for one minute as you take long, deep breaths with your eyes closed.

Slip your shoes off for the next three steps of this routine if you still feel nauseous.

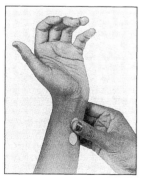

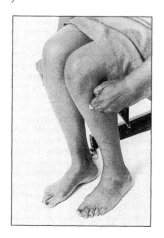

Step 2

Firmly press P 5 and P 6: Place your right thumb on the inside of your left forearm three finger widths from the center of your wrist crease. Apply firm pressure with your thumb for one minute, placing your fingertips directly behind as you take a few long, deep breaths. Then place your thumb two finger widths from your wrist crease and apply pressure for another minute. Firmly press these points on your other wrist for one minute each as you breathe deeply.

Step 4

Stimulate St 36: Place your right fist on the outside of your right leg and your left fist on the outside of your left leg. Briskly rub up and down beside the shinbone for thirty seconds.

175

Step 5

Rub Lv 3: Place your right heel on the top of your left foot in between the bones that attach to your large and second toes. Use your heel to briskly rub this point for thirty seconds. Then repeat on your other foot.

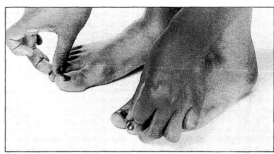

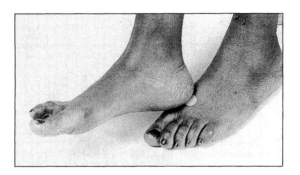

Step 6

Squeeze St 45: Use your thumb and middle finger to firmly squeeze both sides of the base of your second toenail. Hold for thirty seconds on each side.

If you still feel nauseous, a gentle walk, swinging your hands freely by your sides, may help settle your stomach. Don't go to bed — it makes things worse. Try to keep moving in cold, fresh air.

Additional Points for Relieving Nausea

For illustrations of related points for relieving motion sickness, morning sickness, and nausea, see chapter 39, "Stomachaches, Indigestion, and Heartburn."

33

NECK TENSION AND PAIN

*B*ecause the neck is located between the mind and the body, it tends to register conflicts between them, resulting in neck pain or tension. Neck tension tends to accumulate when the needs of either the body or the mind are neglected, creating an energy imbalance. For instance, your body may be tired and need to relax, but your mind may think that you should work. This type of mind-body conflict commonly yields neck tension, as do others such as excessive concentration on material and intellectual pursuits at the expense of the spiritual and emotional dimensions of our lives.

Whenever the neck is strained, it has difficulty properly supporting the head, which weighs about ten to fifteen pounds. Emotional stress and strain create an additional burden on the neck muscles and create even more tension. Because many people do not know how to relieve this tension, it builds and can become chronic. Neck tension, pain, stiffness, and even pinched nerves in the neck are all too common.

The neck is also a barometer for self-expression and change. It is the center from which we vocally express our feelings, thoughts, hopes, and plans. One way to prevent neck tension is to express yourself appropriately and try to maintain a harmonious balance within yourself. Unfortunately, we are constantly being challenged to make changes in relation to the dynamics and transitions of life, so we probably will always have some neck tension!

Whiplash

The violent impact of a car accident can traumatize the neck muscles and vertebrae. A whiplash can create many long term problems such as headaches, neck pain and stiffness, shoulder problems, insomnia, numbness in the arms, and ringing in the ears.

After an accident, a physician should carefully examine the injuries to determine what damage has occurred. Once any inflammation subsides, gentle acupressure can be beneficial to increase circulation and promote healing.

People who have had whiplashes months or even years earlier and who still suffer from the injury can benefit greatly from acupressure. Once the effects of the injury become chronic, it's necessary to apply acupressure once or twice a day for several months to achieve maximum results. The lead singer of one of my favorite local musical groups had severe neck pain due to two automobile accidents. After she had pressed points on her shoulders and neck regularly for three weeks, she said she felt free of pain for the first time in two years.

Potent Points for Relieving Neck Tension and Pain

Shoulder Well (GB 21)

Caution: Press lightly on pregnant women.

Location: On the highest point of the shoulder, one to two inches out from the base of the neck on the tightest spot.

Benefits: Relieves stiff neck, irritability, shoulder tension, and poor circulation.

Heavenly Pillar (B 10)

Location: One-half inch below the base of the skull, on the ropy muscles one-half inch outward from the spine.

Benefits: Relieves stress, exhaustion, stiff necks, and sore throats.

Gates of Consciousness (GB 20)

Location: Below the base of the skull, in the hollows that lie approximately two to three inches apart, depending on the size of the head.

Benefits: Relieves stiff necks, neck pain, arthritis in the neck, and headaches.

Window of Heaven (TW 16)

Location: In the indentation at the base of the skull, one to two inches in back of the earlobe, depending on the size of the head.

Benefits: Relieves stiff necks, shoulder and neck pain, and headaches.

Wind Mansion (GV 16)

Location: In the center of the back of the head in the large hollow under the base of the skull.

Benefits: Good for the eyes, ears, nose, and throat. Relieves headaches, vertigo, stiff necks, and neck pain.

Drilling Bamboo (B 2)

Location: In the indentation of the inner eye socket, where the bridge of the nose meets the ridge of the eyebrows.

Benefits: Relieves neck pain, headaches, hay fever, eye fatigue, and pain in general.

■ *You do not have to use all of these points. Using just one or two of them whenever you have a free hand can be effective.*

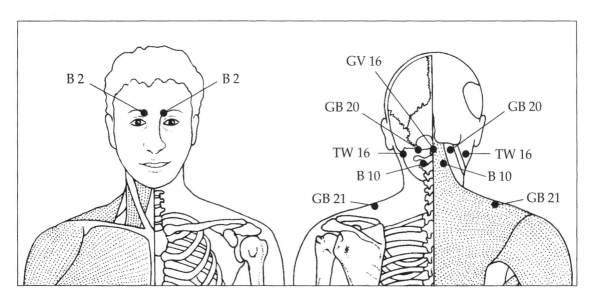

Potent Point Exercises

The following acupressure routine, which can be practiced sitting or lying down, helps keep the neck flexible and strong, and relieves neck pain and tension.

Step 1

Grasp GB 21: Curve your fingers of both hands and place them on the tops of your shoulder muscles close to the base of your neck. Gradually apply firm pressure directly on your shoulder tension. Simply let the weight of your arms relax forward, keeping your fingers curved like a hook. Sink deeper into the muscles as they soften and relax.

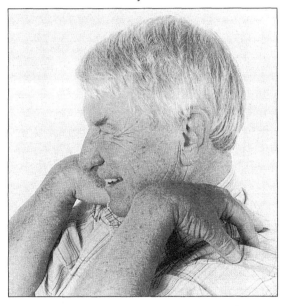

Hold for one minute as you take long, slow, deep breaths. Then let your hands relax in your lap, and shrug your shoulders up and down several times to let them completely relax.

Step 2

Firmly press B 10: Again, curve your fingers and place all of your fingertips on the thick, ropy muscles on the back of your neck.

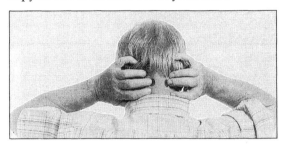

Continue to apply firm pressure on these muscles as you slowly move your head up and down for one minute. Inhale as you raise your head up and back, and exhale as you let your head come forward. Maintain firm pressure as you repeat this movement several times, breathing deeply all the while.

Step 3

Press GB 20 and TW 16: Place your thumbs underneath the base of your skull in the indentations that lie about two to three inches apart. Close your eyes and gradually press up under the skull for at least one minute. Then slide your thumbs outward to TW 16 in the indentations behind your earlobes. Because this point is often sensitive, use care to apply the pressure gradually upward into the base of the skull. Hold this point for another minute as you breathe deeply.

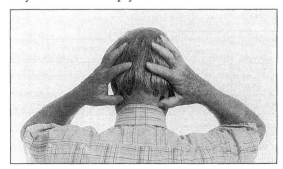

Step 4

Hold GV 16 with B 2: Place your left thumb in the large hollow underneath the center of your skull. Use your thumb and index finger of your right hand to grasp the upper eye sockets, near the bridge of your nose. Squeeze your thumb and index finger together as you press upward. Breathe slowly and deeply as you hold this point combination for one minute.

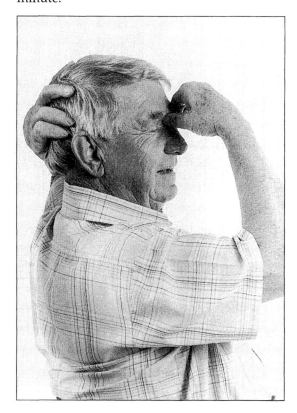

Neck Press Exercise

Interlace your fingers together at the back of your neck and let your head hang forward,

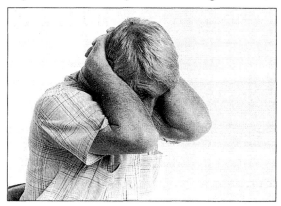

with your elbows close together and pointing down toward your lap. Inhale deeply, raising your head as you stretch your elbows out to the sides; let your head tilt back. Exhale as your head relaxes forward and your elbows come close together in front of you. Repeat this exercise for one to two minutes, then let your hands float back into your lap. Take another minute with your eyes closed to feel yourself relax.

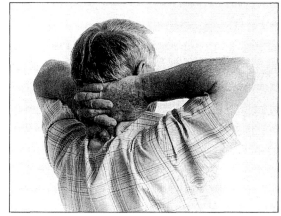

Additional Points for Relieving Neck Tension and Pain

For illustrations of other related points for relieving neck tension and pain, see chapter 11, "Colds and Flu"; chapter 20, "Headaches and Migraines"; and chapter 35, "Pain."

34
Nosebleeds

*G*eneral stress, trauma, and dryness can be contributing causes of a nosebleed. But if nosebleeding recurs frequently or regularly, it may be a symptom of a more complex illness such as high blood pressure, hypertension, leukemia, or arteriosclerosis, all of which require medical attention.

Acupressure, along with direct pressure such as plugging the nose with sterile cotton and keeping the head up as high as possible, can be especially helpful. Ice packs can also be used in severe cases to inhibit nosebleeding. Because stress can unbalance the autonomic nervous system and cause many nosebleeds, make sure you are completely relaxed as you hold the acupressure points. These points are safe and useful to teach your child.

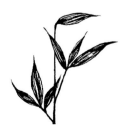

Potent Points for Relieving Nosebleeds

Middle of a Person (GV 26)

Location: Two-thirds the way up from the upper lip to the nose.

Benefits: This first-aid revival point has traditionally been used for relieving nosebleeds, muscle cramps, fainting, and dizziness.

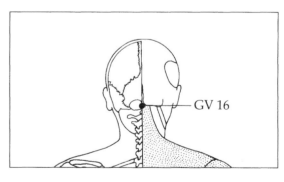
Back of hand

Joining the Valley (Hoku) (LI 4)

Caution: This point is forbidden for pregnant women until labor because its stimulation can cause premature contractions in the uterus.

Location: In the webbing between the thumb and index finger at the highest spot of the muscle when the thumb and index finger are brought close together.

Benefits: Relieves sinus pain, nosebleeds, hay fever, headaches, and toothaches.

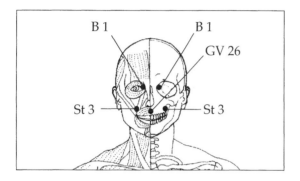

Facial Beauty (St 3)

Location: At the bottom of the cheekbone, directly below the pupil of the eye.

Benefits: Relieves sinus pain, eye fatigue, and pressure as well as nasal and head congestion.

Eyes Bright (B 1)

Location: In the hollow at the inner corner of the eye just above the tear duct.

Benefits: First aid acupressure point for severe nosebleeds. Also relieves eye pain.

■ *You do not have to use all of these points. Using just one or two of them whenever you have a free hand can be effective.*

Wind Mansion (GV 16)

Location: In the center of the back of the head in the large hollow under the base of the skull.

Benefits: Good for the eyes, ears, nose, and throat. Relieves headaches, stiff necks, nosebleeds, and neck pain.

Potent Point Exercises

The following self-acupressure routine for relieving nosebleeds can be practiced lying down on your back or sitting up with your head tilted back.

Step 3

Grasp LI 4: Spread your thumb and index finger apart as you press into the muscle of the web for one minute. Then press the webbing of your other hand for another minute.

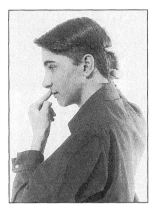

Step 1

Press GV 26 with GV 16: When a nosebleed starts, immediately press GV 26 (below the tip of the nose) using firm pressure on the upper gum. Use your other hand to hold GV 16, in the large hollow under the center of the base of the skull, for one minute as you breathe deeply.

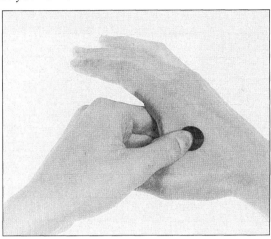

Step 2

Hold both St 3 points: Use your index fingers to lightly press upward into a slight hollow underneath the cheekbone for another minute, letting each deep breath relax you.

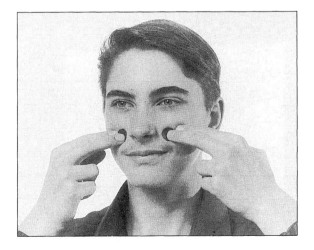

Additional Points for Relieving Nosebleeds

For illustrations of other related points for relieving nosebleeds, see chapter 38, "Sinus Problems and Hay Fever."

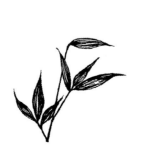

35
PAIN

*P*ain is a red flag indicating that the body needs attention and severe pain is always a sign that you should immediately seek medical assistance. The cause of pain can be physical, emotional, or spiritual. Whatever its basis, though, pain is exacerbated by tension, fatigue, and anxiety. The more tense you are, the more sharply you experience any pain you may be feeling. Stress can also cause neuro-muscular imbalances that can flare up into such painful conditions as backaches or headaches. By relieving tension and increas-ing circulation, acupressure reduces and even prevents pain, while at the same time promot-ing relaxation and healing.

Acupressure can also block the transmis-sion of pain impulses by closing the gates of the body's pain-signaling system and releas-ing endorphins — the neurochemicals that naturally reduce pain without any of the side effects of drugs.

One of my acupressure students who used to be a professional house painter had been suffering from intense nerve pain in his lower back for two days. He'd had a lower-back problem ever since a work injury, when he fell through a roof. Whenever he does hard physical work, his sacroiliac joint goes out of place, and pain extends down the back of his leg. Six weeks earlier, he had also been in a minor car accident and had suffered some whiplash. I showed him how he could use the acupressure points for general pain, which helped him completely relax and take some of the tension out of his muscles and frame. The self-acupressure particularly helped him to have a good night's sleep.

Jerry, a client, was suffering from almost constant pain in his hip and upper back,

which were possible early signs of arthritis. More than five years ago he had been thrown from a horse, which had damaged his spine, although it had long since healed. Because Jerry was in so much pain, he was unable to sleep much at night. He was unable to lie down in bed, and slept only lightly in a recliner. He looked ten years older than his age, with deep furrows between his eyebrows.

I massaged Jerry's hands and feet because there are particularly potent points between the fingers and toes for relieving upper body pain and shoulder tension. Then I showed him points in his shoulder area, working around each wing bone (scapula), down each arm and hand, ending with the pain relief points in the webbing between the thumb and index finger. I also held points on his upper back, shoulders, and neck.

The next week Jerry came into my office standing up straight, looking rested and smiling. He said that it had been years since he slept so soundly on his back. Jerry re-ported that by pressing the acupressure point LI 4, between his thumb and index finger, he was able to relieve his pain immediately.

Hoku, or Joining the Valley (LI 4), is the most widely used point for relieving general pain (this point is described and illustrated fully on the next page). *You can relieve joint and muscular pain anywhere in the body with just this one point!* LI 4 is most effective when used in conjunction with movement. First, isolate the sorest spot in the Hoku area. Hold it firmly enough to produce mild pain. Then move the joint nearest the part of your body that's in pain. If you have a stiff neck, for instance, move your head up and down as you firmly press Hoku. After a minute or two, switch hands to work on the Hoku point on the other side. Again, move the joint that is closest to your pain while you firmly press into LI 4 of your other hand. After just a few minutes, you may find that much of your pain is relieved.

The following points are famous in Oriental health care for relieving pain. These points tend to have a stronger influence on relieving pain in either the upper or the lower portion of the body. If you have generalized musculoskeletal pain in your chest or shoulder, use the upper-body pain points. If you feel pain in your groin, genitals, or legs, use the lower-body pain points. But if you have lower-back or abdominal pain, use both the upper- and lower-body pain points.

Acupuncture frequently uses needles in the following points as general anesthesia for pain anywhere in the body.

Potent Points for Relieving Upper-Body Pain

Joining the Valley (Hoku) (LI 4)

Caution: This point is forbidden for pregnant women until labor because its stimulation can cause premature contractions in the uterus.

Location: In the webbing between the thumb and index finger at the highest spot of the muscle when the thumb and index finger are brought close together.

Benefits: Relieves arthritis, constipation, headaches, toothaches, and shoulder pain.

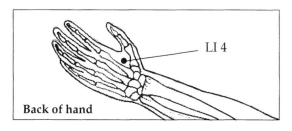

Back of hand

LI 4

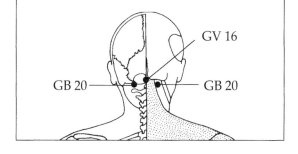

GV 16

GB 20

GB 20

Gates of Consciousness (GB 20)

Location: Below the base of the skull, in the hollows on either side, two to three inches apart depending on the size of the head.

Benefits: Relieves arthritis, headaches, stiff necks, neck pain, and trauma.

Wind Mansion (GV 16)

Location: In the lower center of the back of the head in a large hollow under the base of the skull.

Benefits: Relieves pain in the eyes, ears, nose, and throat. Also relieves headaches and stiff necks.

Third Eye Point

(GV 24.5)

Location: Directly between the eyebrows, in the indentation where the bridge of the nose meets the forehead.

Benefits: This helps the endocrine system, especially the pituitary gland, and relieves hay fever, headaches, and eyestrain.

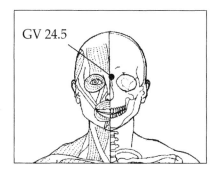

GV 24.5

■ *You do not have to use all of these points. Using just one or two of them whenever you have a free hand can be effective.*

Potent Point Exercises

Step 1

Squeeze LI 4: Firmly press into the webbing between your thumb and index finger for one

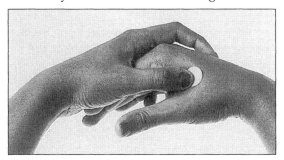

minute. Direct your finger pressure underneath the bone that connects with your index finger. Then switch hands to press on the other LI 4 point for another minute.

Step 2

Firmly press GB 20: Place your thumbs underneath the base of your skull in the hollows that lie about three inches apart.

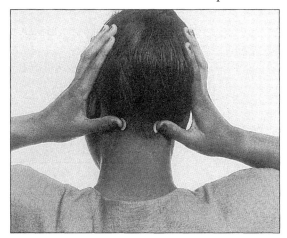

Apply pressure gradually underneath the base of your skull as you slowly tilt your head back. Breathe deeply as you apply firm pressure toward the center of your head for one full minute or until you can feel a regular, even pulse on both sides.

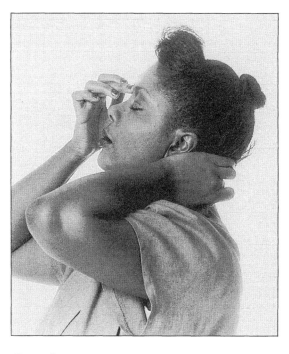

Step 3

Press GV 16 along with the GV 24.5: Place the middle finger of your left hand on GV 16 in the center of the base of your skull. Use the third finger of your right hand to apply light pressure on GV 24.5 in the indentation in between your eyebrows. Close your eyes, slowly tilting your head back, and breathe deeply for one full minute as you focus your attention at that spot. This is an excellent acupressure combination to use when you're having difficulty sleeping due to discomfort or pain.

Potent Points for Relieving Lower-Body Pain

Gates of Consciousness (GB 20)

Location: Below the base of the skull, in the hollows on either side, two to three inches apart depending on the size of the head.

Benefits: Relieves pain in all areas of the body, throbbing headaches, dizziness, stiff neck, coordination problems, and irritability.

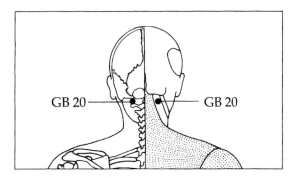

Three Mile Point (St 36)

Location: Four finger widths below the kneecap, one finger width outside of the shinbone. If you are on the correct spot, a muscle should flex as you move your foot up and down.

Benefits: Strengthens the whole body, tones the muscles, aids digestion, and relieves stomach disorders, knee pain, and shin splints.

■ *You do not have to use all of these points. Using just one or two of them can be effective.*

Bigger Stream (K 3)

This point is good for pain in a wisdom tooth.

Caution: Do not stimulate this point after the third month of pregnancy.

Location: Midway between the inside ankle-bone and the Achilles tendon in the back of the ankle.

Benefits: Relieves swollen feet, ankle pain, menstrual cramps, earaches, ringing in the ears, and back pain.

High Mountains (B 60)

Location: Midway between the back edge of the outer anklebone and the Achilles tendon.

Benefits: Relieves sciatica, thigh pain, head-ache, lower-back aches, and rheumatism.

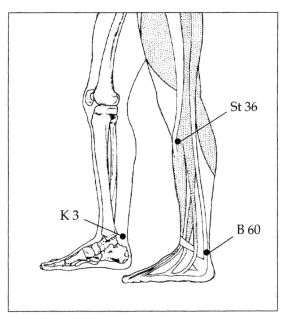

Potent Point Exercises

Step 1

Firmly press GB 20: Place your thumbs underneath the base of your skull in the

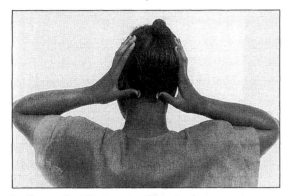

hollows that lie two to three inches apart depending on the size of your head. Apply pressure gradually underneath the base of your skull as you slowly tilt your head back. Breathe deeply for one full minute as you direct firm pressure toward the center of your forehead.

Step 3

Grasp K 3 and B 60: Bend your left leg, placing your left foot on your right knee. Use your right thumb to press K 3, between the inside anklebone and the Achilles tendon. Place your middle and index fingers of your right hand directly in back of your thumb on B

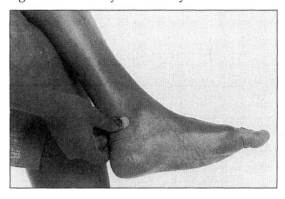

60. Grasp these points with steady, firm pressure for two minutes. Then do the same on the other side.

Step 2

Briskly rub St 36: Measure four finger widths below your kneecap, placing your finger-tips one-half inch outside the shinbone. If you're on the correct spot, a muscle should flex as you move your foot up and down. Now make fists and place them on St 36 on the outside of both legs just below your knees. Use your fists to briskly massage up and down along the outside of your shinbones. Breathe deeply as you briskly rub this point for 1 minute.

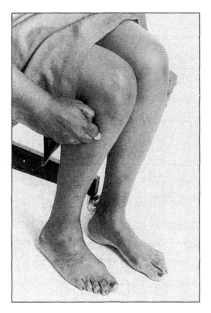

Additional Points for Relieving Pain

For illustrations of other related points for relieving general pain, see chapter 5, "Ankle and Foot Problems"; chapter 6, "Anxiety and Nervousness"; chapter 9, "Backache and Sciatica"; chapter 28, "Knee Pain"; chapter 33, "Neck Tension and Pain"; chapter 41, "Toothaches"; and chapter 42, "Wrist Pain."

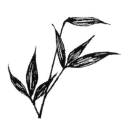

36

PREGNANCY AND INFERTILITY

Some of my most rewarding experiences practicing acupressure has been working with pregnant women. I have shown many women how to relieve the lower-back pain, shoulder, and neck pains that often accompany pregnancy, and I have taught their mates how to help them ease these tensions as well as labor pains.

I have also used acupressure to help women who had difficulty getting pregnant become fertile. One of my recent acupressure graduates gave a session to a client of hers, a female attorney who had tried to become pregnant for two years. This woman and her husband wanted desperately to have a child. She received weekly acupressure sessions that focused on releasing tension in her neck, chest, lower back, and hips. The Hara (CV 6), a

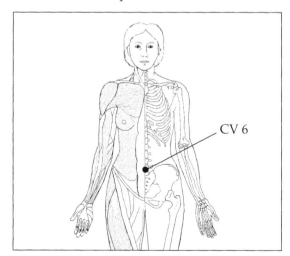

CV 6

special point for toning the abdominal region and for enhancing fertility, was consistently used each week. She also used this point (three finger widths below the belly button) every day for self-treatment. After three

months, she ecstatically reported to her acupressurist that she finally became pregnant.

During pregnancy many physical changes occur within a woman's body. At each stage of pregnancy, specific symptoms occur in response to stresses on the body. For instance, the increase in the size of the fetus puts increasing pressure on the bladder. This creates the need to urinate more frequently. Such powerful physiological changes can be harmonized through the stimulation of appropriate acupressure points. There are points that rebalance the female hormonal system, and points that relieve morning sickness, lower-back aches, swollen ankles, and fatigue.

During the first trimester the most common discomforts are breast tenderness, nausea, and fatigue. Because the acupressure points for relieving breast tenderness are the same points that are used to help with breast-feeding, you should also refer to chapter 29.

To relieve morning sickness, firmly press the inside of your wrist (P 6), which is described and illustrated in the following pages. In fact, this point can be quite effective for relieving all types of nausea, from morning sickness to motion sickness (see chapter 32).

To combat fatigue, stimulate the Sea of Vitality Points, B 23 and B 47, on your lower back. Either rub your lower back briskly with the backs of your hands, using the friction to create heat; or roll up a couple of thick towels, place them under your lower back, and slowly lie down on them to apply pressure to the lower back. These points are effective for relieving fatigue and lower-back strain during pregnancy.

The groin points relieve abdominal pain, indigestion, bloating, and breathing difficulties caused by the fetus moving and placing pressure on the mother's solar plexus. These points (Sp 12 and Sp 13) are located in the pelvic area, where the leg meets the trunk of the body. They are midway between the base of the hipbone and pubic bone. The Womb and Vitals point (described below) relieves pelvic and lower-back tensions, areas that can get blocked, especially during pregnancy, labor, and postpartum recovery.

Caution: Traditionally, using acupuncture needles during pregnancy is forbidden, because strong stimulation of these points can encourage uterine contractions, thus increasing the risk of miscarriage. Acupressure is considered safe, however, though finger pressure on any point during pregnancy should be gradual and moderate. Before trying any of these exercises, check with your doctor to make sure he or she sees no contraindications for their use.

Point	Strong Stimulation Discouraged After	Illustrated on Page
LI 4*	1st Month	186
K 3**	3rd Month	188
Sp 6***	7th Month	169

* Can induce labor
** Calms the fetus.
*** Can induce labor and calms the fetus.

Potent Points for Relieving Discomforts Due to Pregnancy

Sea of Vitality (B 23 and B 47)

Caution: Do not press on disintegrating discs or fractured or broken bones. If you have a weak back, a few minutes of stationary, light touching instead of pressure can be very healing. See your doctor first if you have any questions or need medical advice.

Location: In the lower back two to four finger widths away from the spine at waist level.

Benefits: Relieves postpartum discomforts, lower backaches, fatigue, sexual-reproductive problems, irregular vaginal discharge.

Womb and Vitals (B 48)

Location: One to two finger widths outside the sacrum (the large bony area at the base of the spine) and midway between the top of the hipbone (the iliac crest) and the base of the buttock.

Benefits: Relieves pelvic tension as well as constipation, urinary problems, sciatica, lower-back aches, and hip pain during pregnancy.

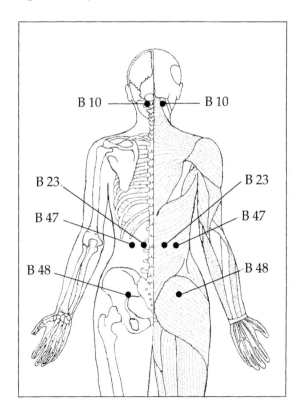

Heavenly Pillar (B 10)

Location: One-half inch below the base of the skull, on the ropy muscles one-half inch outward from the spine.

Benefits: Relieves the following common complaints during pregnancy: stress, exhaustion, insomnia, head congestion, stiff neck, and swollen eyes.

Sea of Tranquility (CV 17)

Location: On the center of the breastbone, three thumb widths up from the base of the bone.

Benefits: Relieves nervousness, chest congestion, insomnia, anxiety, depression, and other emotional imbalances during pregnancy.

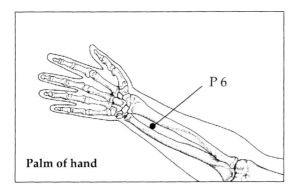

Palm of hand

Inner Gate (P 6)

Location: In the middle of the inner side of the forearm two-and-one-half finger widths below the wrist crease.

Benefits: Relieves discomforts during pregnancy and postpartum, nausea, insomnia, anxiety, and indigestion.

■ *You do not have to use all of these points. Using just one or two of them whenever you have a free hand can be effective.*

Third Eye Point (GV 24.5)

Location: Directly between the eyebrows, in the indentation where the bridge of the nose meets the forehead.

Benefits: Regulates glandular imbalances during pregnancy and relieves hay fever, headaches, and indigestion.

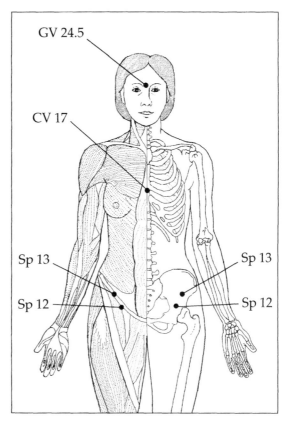

Rushing Door (Sp 12)
Mansion Cottage (Sp 13)

These two points are effective for releasing abdominal discomforts during pregnancy.

Location: Both points are in the pelvic area in the middle of the crease where the leg joins the trunk of the body.

Benefits: These points are particularly good for relieving impotency, menstrual cramps, and abdominal discomfort.

Potent Point Exercises

Although you can use these points individually in any position, this routine is designed to be practiced lying down comfortably on your back in bed or on a carpeted floor.

Step 1

Stimulate the B 48 area: With your legs bent and your feet flat on the floor, place your hands underneath your buttocks (with your

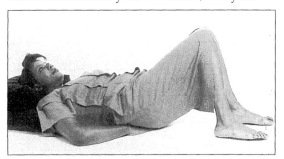

palms down) beside the base of your spine. Take long, deep breaths as you sway your knees from side to side for two minutes. Reposition your hands for comfort and to press different parts of the buttock muscles.

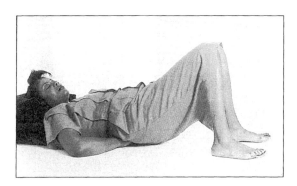

Step 2

Press B 23 and B 47: Use a tightly rolled up pair of thick socks or make fists with your knuckles facing up. Arch your pelvis upward, lifting your buttocks off the ground to position

the socks or the knuckles of your fist four inches apart underneath your lower back, at the level of your waist. Slowly lower your buttocks to the floor, letting yourself relax as you take long, slow, deep breaths for one minute. This will put pressure on both the inner and outer lower back points. Then lift your pelvis up again, bringing the socks or your hands out from underneath you, and let your hands relax by your sides. Now lower your pelvis back down to the floor and completely relax.

Step 3

Firmly press B 10: Place the fingertips of both hands on the back of the neck one-half inch out from of the spine on either side. Use all of your fingertips to firmly press the thick, ropy muscles that run parallel to the spine. With the backs of your hands on the floor and your fingers curved, firmly lift up your neck muscles for one full minute as you breathe deeply.

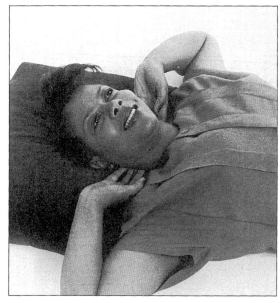

Step 4

Press P 6: Place your right thumb on the inside of your left wrist, two-and-one-half finger widths below the center of your wrist crease. Press firmly and hold for thirty seconds. Then switch hands to press your right wrist, holding for another thirty seconds.

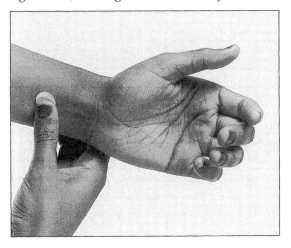

Step 5

Hold GV 24.5 with CV 17: Gently place the third finger of your right hand between your eyebrows on the Third Eye Point. Use the fingertips of your left hand to hold the indentations on the center of your breastbone. Hold this calming potent point combination for at least one minute as you breathe deeply.

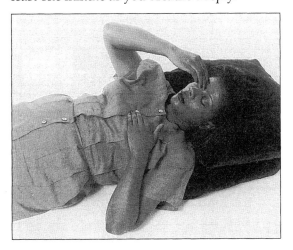

Special Pregnancy Lower-Back Release

Lay two towels out flat, one on top of the other. Fold the outer edges of the towel in toward the center. Roll the towel up tightly and place it on a carpeted floor. Lie down on your back with the towels underneath the base of your spine. Your legs can be bent or straight, whichever is most comfortable.

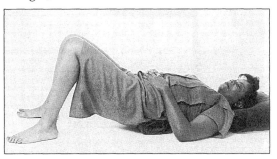

Place your hands on your belly, close your eyes, and breathe deeply for at least two minutes. Then bend your knees with your feet flat on the floor and arch your pelvis up to bring the towel out from underneath you. Lower your buttocks down to the floor and let yourself completely relax with your eyes closed for several minutes.

As you breathe deeply into your womb, visualize each breath nourishing your baby. Let all the love in your heart connect with your womb and let yourself completely relax.

Additional Points for Pregnancy and Infertility

For illustrations of other related points for relieving discomfort during pregnancy, see chapter 29, "Labor, Delivery, and Nursing."

37

SHOULDER TENSION

Sally, my mother's best friend, suffered from shoulder bursitis and upper arm pain. Her upper back was also quite tender. I gave her about half an hour of acupressure on her shoulders and showed her how to press the points on herself. Much to our mutual surprise, Sally was immediately able to raise her upper arm without pain. She later reported that her pain returned occasionally, but that now she was able to relieve it simply by holding the points on herself.

Pain or tightness in the shoulder area often reflects a person's overall emotional and physical state. A stressful lifestyle, emotional strains, physical injuries, and fatigue can contribute to constriction and pain in the shoulders.

Many occupations also create and reinforce shoulder tensions. Typing, working at a desk, or working at a machine or computer can cause shoulder tension. When you slump, your breathing gets shallow, and tensions develop. Truck drivers who hunch their shoulders as they hold the wheel develop these tensions. People who do highly detailed, close work such as electronics, graphic arts, needlework, or jewelry making have a similar problem. Anyone in competitive, stressful situations, whether an executive or a student, can suffer from shoulder tension.

The shoulders are the repository for much of our tension and stress. Eventually the tension becomes chronic, contributing to fatigue, and that affects other parts of the body. Chronic shoulder tension can inhibit the circulation to the extremities, causing cold hands and feet. By releasing shoulder tension, a wave of warmth can be released into the arms and hands; some people report greater circulation in their legs and feet as well.

Acupressure is effective for relieving both shoulder and neck tension. When you practice on yourself, it usually takes several applications (fifteen to twenty minutes) of finger pressure along with deep breathing to alleviate shoulder pain or a stiff neck. Often you will find great relief in your shoulders each time you apply acupressure to yourself. But because shoulder problems are often an accumulation of various tensions or injuries over a period of months (maybe even years), it normally takes several acupressure sessions to completely release them.

This chapter covers specific local acupressure points on the shoulders as well as trigger points located farther away from the area that nonetheless release shoulder pain and stiffness. Several minutes of firm pressure on the Heavenly Rejuvenation point (TW 15) relieves shoulder pain and tension as well as stiff necks. GB 21 is another major point where shoulder tension collects. It is located on the top of the shoulder muscle near the base of the neck. LI 14 (on the upper arm) and GB 20 (at the base of the skull) are excellent trigger points for relieving shoulder pain and chronic tension. These points, described here, are all suitable for teaching to children.

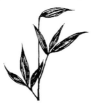

Potent Points for Relieving Shoulder Tension

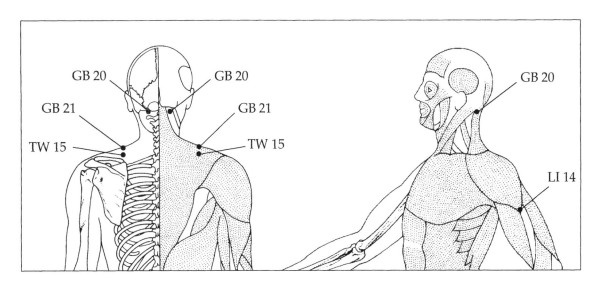

Heavenly Rejuvenation (TW 15)

Location: On the shoulders, midway between the base of the neck and the outside of the shoulders, one-half inch below the top of the shoulders.

Benefits: Relieves muscular tension, stiff necks, and shoulder pain.

Shoulder Well (GB 21)

Caution: Pregnant women should press lightly on this point.

Location: On the muscle at the highest point of the shoulder, one to two inches out from the side of the lower neck.

Benefits: Relieves shoulder tension, nervousness, irritability, and fatigue.

Outer Arm Bone (LI 14)

Location: On the outer surface of the upper arm one-third of the way down from the top of the shoulder to the elbow. Find a wiry muscle band by rubbing the fingers over the bone on the outside of the arm.

Benefits: Relieves aching in the arm, shoulder tension, and stiff necks.

Gates of Consciousness (GB 20)

Location: Below the base of the skull, in the hollow between the two large vertical neck muscles, two to three inches apart depending on the size of the head.

Benefits: Relieves arthritis in the shoulders and neck, headaches, and stiff neck.

■ *You do not have to use all of these points. Using just one or two of them whenever you have a free hand can be effective.*

Potent Point Exercises

Practice the following routine sitting comfortably.

Step 1

Gently pound your shoulders: Make a loose fist with your right hand, keeping your wrist loose. Use the fist to pat your left shoulder lightly, tapping the side of your neck, across your chest, and back to the shoulder. Then switch sides and work on your other shoulder. Be sure to spend more time and attention on the side that feels tightest.

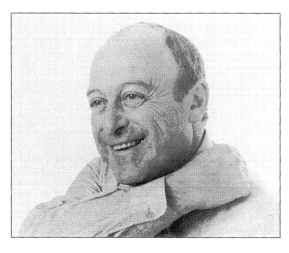

Step 2

Firmly hook into TW 15: Curve your fingers on both hands and place them over the tops of your shoulders, your right hand on your right shoulder, your left hand on your left shoulder. Feel for a marble of tension directly above the top of the shoulder blade.

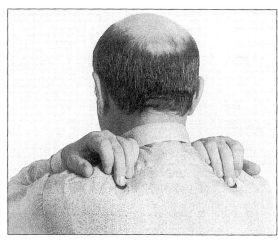

Press the tightest spot on your shoulders with your index, middle, and ring fingers. Allow the weight of your arms to relax forward with your fingers hooked onto the shoulder tension. Breathe deeply as you hold this point for one minute.

Step 3

Hold GB 21 with LI 14: Place your right index, middle, and ring fingertips on the top

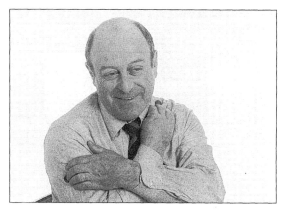

of your left shoulder (GB 21), and your left fingertips on the outside of your right upper arm (LI 14) and press both points. This is a powerful combination for relieving chronic shoulder tension. Hold these potent points for one minute as you take long, deep breaths. Gradually press deeper into the shoulder muscle as it softens and relaxes. Then switch sides, holding for another minute as you continue to breathe deeply.

Step 4

Press GB 20: Place your thumbs underneath the base of your skull, in the indentations that lie two to three inches apart. Slowly tilt your head back as you gradually press up and under the skull with your eyes closed. Take long, deep breaths as you direct the pressure firmly up under the skull and inward. Take long, slow, deep breaths as you hold this point for one minute or until you feel a regular, even pulse on both sides. Then very slowly release the pressure.

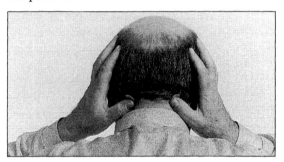

Shoulder Grasp and Pull

Curve the fingers of your right hand over your left shoulder, hooking them into the tight (trapezius) muscle. Inhale as you gradually apply firm pressure with your fingers; hold for a few seconds and exhale, slowly raking your fingers up and over your shoulder, firmly stretching the muscle. Then let your right hand fall back into your lap. Next, work on your right shoulder. Using your left hand, hook your fingers firmly into the muscle on the top of your right shoulder and repeat the movements. Inhale deeply as you apply firm,

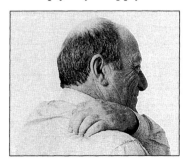

steady pressure with your fingers. Hold. And exhale slowly, raking your fingers over your shoulder, giving a nice, firm stretch to that muscle. Then let your left hand float into your lap. Breathe deeply as you relax.

Acu-Yoga Exercise for Releasing Shoulder Tension

In the following exercise your body will be positioned so that your weight presses the muscles and points on your shoulders to relieve the tension there. This posture is most effective when you concentrate on breathing deeply. It is good for relieving shoulder tension, frustration and irritability.

1. Lie on your back.
2. Bend your knees so that the soles of your feet are flat on the floor.
3. Put your arms above your head on the floor and relax them.
4. Inhale, arching the pelvis up; hold for several seconds.

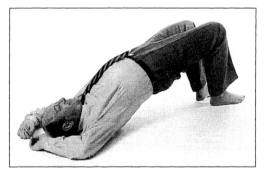

5. Exhale as you slowly come down; continue to inhale as you move up and exhale as you move down for one minute.
6. Relax on your back with your hands by your sides and your eyes closed for a few minutes and continue to breathe deeply.

Additional Points for Releasing Shoulder Tension

For other related points to relieve shoulder tension, see chapter 26, "Irritability, Frustration, and Dealing with Change"; and chapter 33, "Neck Tension and Pain."

38

SINUS PROBLEMS AND HAY FEVER

*A*lthough acupressure techniques relieve sinus conditions, it is imperative to go beyond relieving the symptoms to discover and eliminate the causes of the problem. If you have chronic problems with your sinuses, consult your doctor. In many cases, sinus problems can be the result of strong emotions, such as worry, grief, or guilt. When these feelings are unresolved they often cause muscular tension in the chest, which also tends to close the sinus passages. As acupressure releases this tension, the sinuses often clear.

Constipation, a poor diet, or lack of exercise can contribute to sinus problems. To see if your diet is affecting your sinuses, unless your physician advises against it, try to abstain from all dairy products for two weeks, and see if your sinus condition improves.

Dennis, a former client, used acupressure points beside his nose to relieve chronic nasal congestion and restore his sense of smell. He used these points several times each day for two weeks, and discovered that his sense of taste also improved.

Structurally, the sinuses resemble pockets or valleys. The acupressure point that is traditionally recommended for treatment of hay fever and the sinuses is LI 4, Joining the Valley. As a trigger point for relieving general congestion and pain, LI 4 helps open up and drain the sinuses. B 2 at the bridge of the nose is helpful for frontal headaches and sinus conditions. On the skull, the GV 20 and B 7 points have also traditionally been used to help open up congested nasal passages. LI 20 and St 3 on the face are the foremost points for dealing with the maxillary sinuses located in the cheek area. These points are safe and useful to teach to children.

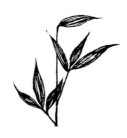

Potent Points for Relieving Sinus and Hay Fever Problems

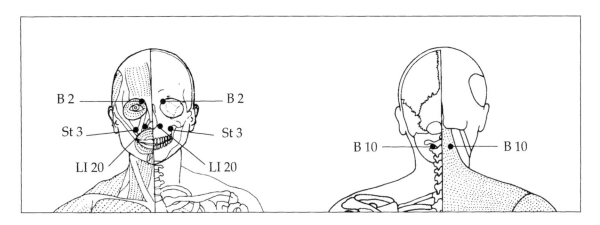

Drilling Bamboo (B 2)

Location: In the indentation of the inner eye socket where the bridge of the nose meets the ridge of the eyebrows.

Benefits: Relieves sinus pain, headaches, blurry vision, red and watery eyes, hay fever, and eyestrain.

Heavenly Pillar (B 10)

Location: One-half inch below the base of the skull on the ropy muscles one-half inch outward from the spine.

Benefits: Relieves head congestion, hay fever, stress, burnout, stiff necks, swollen eyes, and sore throats.

Penetrate Heaven (B 7)

Location: On the top of the skull, in a line upward from the back of the ears, one thumb width from the center.

Benefits: Relieves headaches, stuffy nose, sinus and head congestion, and a weak sense of smell.

Welcoming Perfume (LI 20)

Location: Just to the side of the nostril.

Benefits: Relieves sinus pain, nasal congestion, facial paralysis, and facial swelling.

Facial Beauty (St 3)

Location: At the bottom of the cheekbone, directly below the pupil.

Benefits: Relieves stuffy nose, head congestion, burning eyes, toothaches, and eye fatigue.

One Hundred Meeting Point (GV 20)

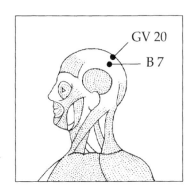

Location: On the crown of the head between the cranial bones. To find the point, follow the line up from the back of the ears to the top of the head.

Benefits: Relieves sinus congestion, poor concentration and memory, and headaches.

Third Eye Point (GV 24.5)

Location: Directly between the eyebrows, in the indentation where the bridge of the nose meets the forehead.

Benefits: Relieves hay fever, sinus congestion, headaches, and eyestrain.

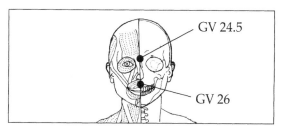

Middle of a Person (GV 26)

Location: Two-thirds of the way up from the upper lip to the nose.

Benefits: Relieves hay fever, sneezing, fainting, and dizziness.

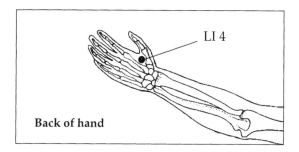

Back of hand

Joining the Valley (Hoku) (LI 4)

Caution: This point is forbidden for pregnant women because its stimulation can cause premature contractions in the uterus.

Location: In the webbing between the thumb and index finger, at the highest spot of the muscle when you bring the thumb and index finger close together.

Benefits: Relieves headaches, sinus pain, and hay fever, as well as head congestion.

■ *You do not have to use all of these points. Using just one or two of them whenever you have a free hand can be effective.*

Potent Point Exercises

Whether you use the following routine for relief or prevention, you can practice it either lying down or sitting comfortably.

Step 1

Firmly press B 2 with B 10: Place your left hand on both B 2 points, near the bridge of the nose, using your thumb on the left side and your index finger on the right . Press up into the slight indentations of the inner, upper eye sockets. Use your right hand to grasp both sides of the back of your neck, using your fingertips on the left side and the heel of your hand on the right side to firmly squeeze your neck muscles. Close your eyes and breathe deeply as you hold these points for at least one minute.

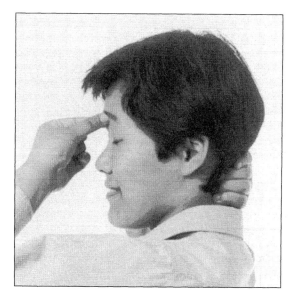

Step 2

Hold B 7: To find this point, place the fingertips of both hands in back of your ears; then move upward to the top of your head. These points are located in the indentations on the top of the head, one inch apart in two slight indentations. Breathe deeply as you hold these points with your fingertips for one minute.

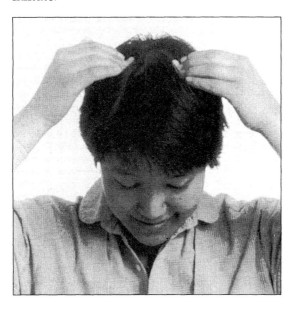

Step 3

Lightly press LI 20 along with St 3: Gently press underneath the cheekbones, beside your nose, angling the pressure upward. Breathe deeply as you hold these points.

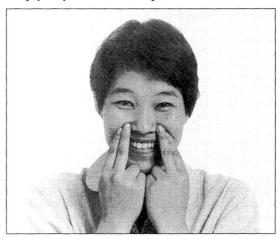

Step 4

Hold GV 20 along with GV 24.5: Place your right fingertips on GV 20 in an indentation on the center top of your head (the baby's soft spot). Use the third fingertip of your left hand to lightly touch in between your eyebrows. Breathe deeply for one minute.

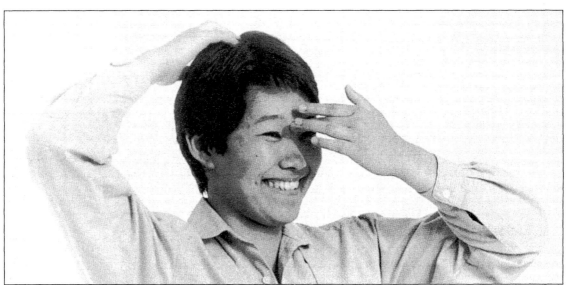

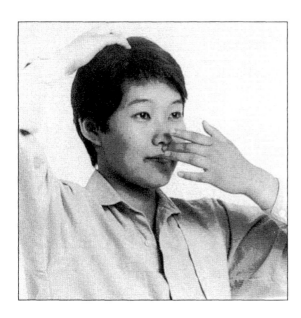

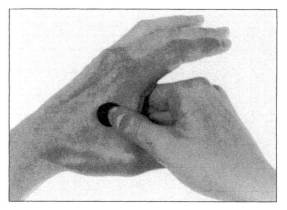

Step 5

Press GV 20 along with GV 26: Continuing to hold GV 20 on the top of the head, move from the Third Eye Point to GV 26 between your upper lip and nose. Breathe deeply as you hold these important potent points firmly for one minute to relieve your hay fever and sinus problems.

Step 6

Firmly grasp LI 4: Place your right thumb in the webbing on the back of your left hand, with your fingers on the palm directly behind your thumb. Squeeze your thumb and index finger together to firmly press into the web-bing. Angle the pressure toward the bone that connects with your left index finger. Take long, slow, deep breaths as you continue to press this point for thirty seconds. Then switch sides to hold your right hand for thirty more seconds. This decongestant trigger point can be used by itself at any time to relieve sinus pain and hay fever.

Additional Points for Relieving Sinus Problems and Hay Fever

For illustrations of other related points for relieving sinus problems and hay fever, see chapter 11, "Colds and Flus"; chapter 20, "Headaches and Migraines"; and chapter 34, "Nosebleeds."

39

STOMACHACHES, INDIGESTION, AND HEARTBURN

*T*here are many causes of stomachaches and indigestion: eating processed foods such as products made with white flour and white sugar; eating rich foods that are difficult to digest, such as heavy sauces, fried foods, and desserts; or overeating or eating foods in improper combinations. Various foods require both different enzymes and different amounts of time to be digested thoroughly. When fruits and beans are eaten together they ferment, causing putrefaction in the digestive system.

Abdominal tension, lack of exercise, or emotional stress can also cause indigestion. Dr. Katsusuke Serizawa of Tokyo University, an authority on Oriental medicine, has found acupressure to be effective in treating indigestion that results from emotional or psychological problems.[41]

When the digestive organs are subject to excess stress and tension, their functioning can be hampered, causing indigestion, abdominal pain, belching, or gas. Tension in the abdominal muscles, the diaphragm, or the digestive organs themselves affects digestion no matter what or how you eat.

Abdominal tensions can produce a deep irritation in the pit of the stomach and sometimes drives a person to overeat unconsciously, in an attempt to relieve that tension. Overeating puts an extra burden on the digestive system and increases abdominal tensions, further imbalancing digestive mechanisms. The potent points in this chapter can alleviate indigestion and also help you fight the urge to overeat.

Ted, one of my clients, complained of having trouble digesting any solid food. After eating he would have terrible abdominal cramps and indigestion, but two doctors he visited couldn't find anything wrong with him. I showed him how to use an important local point in the pit of the stomach. After a week of practicing acupressure on himself two to three times a day, Ted reported that he was now able to digest most varieties of food.

Shelly, one of my advanced acupressure students, reported she had helped her mother, who suffered from acute stomach pain, recover from two major surgeries: Her gallbladder was removed because of gallstones and twelve inches of her small intestine were also removed. Her posture was stooped, her face was pale, and her voice was weak and quivery. Shelly concentrated on pressing the acupressure points on the lower back and the

---

[41] Katsusuke Serizawa, M.D., *Tsubo: Vital Points for Oriental Therapy* (Tokyo: Japan Publications, 1986), 114.

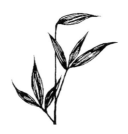

arch of her mother's foot. After forty-five minutes, the bloating in her mother's solar plexus was gone, she felt calmer, the pain in her stomach was relieved, and her face had a healthy glow. The acupressure helped not only her mother's physical pain but also created the bond between mother and daughter. "I felt joy, satisfaction, and wholeness when Mom allowed me to nurture, heal, and give her love . . . this was the most profound experience I have ever had with my mother."

If indigestion or stomachache is severe, see a medical doctor immediately. Appendicitis and a hiatal hernia, for instance, can cause severe abdominal pain and require immediate medical attention. If indigestion or stomachaches occur frequently, you should also consult a physician to see if you have an underlying condition that requires treatment.

The point for relieving abdominal pain and preventing indigestion before you eat is CV 12, located between the navel and the base

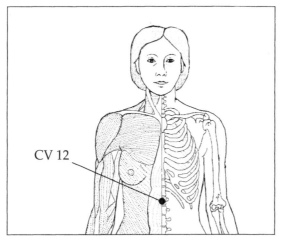

CV 12

of the sternum. It is important to use this point only when your stomach is fairly empty. Wait for two hours after you've eaten before trying it. Lie on your back with your knees bent, feet flat on the floor and your eyes closed, as you gradually press into the pit of the stomach at a forty-five degree angle up toward the diaphragm. Slowly apply pressure on the lump or muscle mass lodged at this abdominal point for about two minutes while

you breathe deeply to release any abdominal tension. When your abdominal muscles are relaxed and balanced, the stomach and intestines are free to function properly. As you breathe fully, the rhythmic movements of the diaphragm massage the stomach internally. You can teach this self-acupressure and breathing exercise to a maturing child over twelve years of age.

Tips for Preventing and Relieving Stomachaches and Indigestion

- **Reduce stomach acidity.** Blend or mash a salt plum[42] in a cup of hot water. This is not to be taken by anybody with high blood pressure.

- **Avoid eating cold foods.** Gulping iced drinks can temporarily paralyze your stomach. Traditional Chinese medicine lists cold foods as one of the major causes of digestive disorders.

- **Relax.** Relaxation before and during eating promotes good digestion. Take several long, slow, deep breaths with your eyes closed before you begin a meal to relieve your stress, instead of repressing it with food.

- **Eat slowly.** Chew your food thoroughly. Hurried eating and incomplete chewing hinder digestion because the enzymes in the saliva that begin the digestive process don't get a chance to do their job. This puts an added burden on the stomach.

- **Try fasting.** Fast for for twenty-four hours with juices, tea, or lemonade. If you start feeling unwell or weak, break the fast early with vegetable soup or steamed vegetables. If you complete the fast, also eat a mild soup or steamed vegetables.

---

[42] Salt plums, or *umeboshi*, are available in most health food stores and Japanese food stores.

Potent Points for Relieving Stomachaches, Indigestion, and Heartburn

Center of Power (CV 12)

Caution: Do not hold this point deeply if you have a chronic or life-threatening illness such as heart disease, cancer, or high blood pressure. (See the caution on page 9.) It is best not to hold this point for more than two minutes and to use it only on a fairly empty stomach.

Location: On the midline of the body, one-half way between the base of the breastbone and the belly button.

Benefits: Relieves stomach pains, abdominal spasms, indigestion, heartburn, constipation, and emotional stress such as worry and frustration that often causes digestive problems.

Sea of Energy (CV 6)

Location: Two finger widths below the navel.

Benefits: Relieves abdominal pain, lower back pain, constipation, gas, and digestive problems.

Sea of Vitality (B 23 and B 47)

Caution: Do not press on disintegrating discs or fractured or broken bones. If you have a weak back, a few minutes of stationary, light touching instead of pressure can be very healing. See your doctor first if you have any questions or need medical advice.

Location: On the lower back two to four finger widths from the spine at waist level.

Benefits: Relieves indigestion, abdominal pain, and stomachaches.

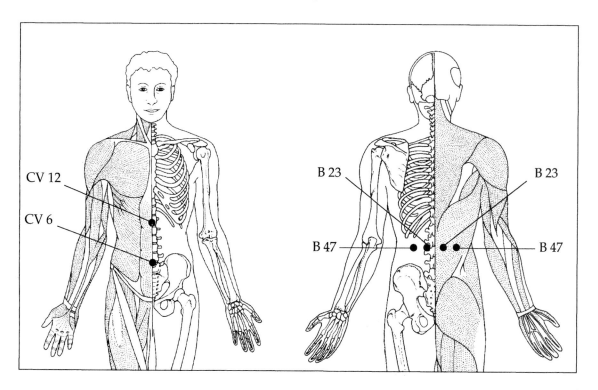

Three Mile Point (St 36)

Location: Four finger widths below the kneecap, one finger width to the outside of the shinbone. If you are on the correct spot, a muscle should flex as you move your foot up and down.

Benefits: Relieves stomachaches, poor digestion, stomach disorders, and fatigue.

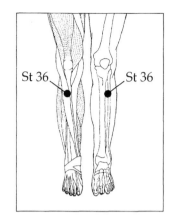

Inner Gate (P 6)

Location: In the middle of the inner wrist, two-and-one-half finger widths below the wrist crease.

Benefits: Relieves stomachaches, indigestion, nausea, and anxiety.

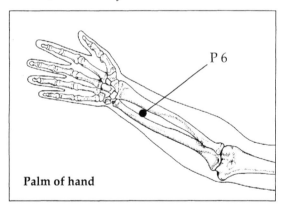

Palm of hand

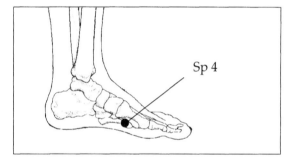

Grandfather Grandson (Sp 4)

Location: On the arch, one thumb width from the ball of the foot toward the heel.

Benefits: Relieves abdominal cramps, stomachaches, indigestion, and diarrhea. Also good for balancing a person who is inclined toward anxiety or hypochondria.

■ *You do not have to use all of these points. Just pressing P 6 firmly for a couple of minutes, whenever you have a free hand, can be effective.*

Potent Point Exercises

If after eating you have an immediate heartburn and find it inappropriate to lie down, use the last three points of this self-acupressure routine: the Inner Gate point (P 6), Three Mile point (St 36), and Grandfather Grandson (Sp 4). The full routine can be practiced on your bed or on a carpeted floor.[43]

Step 1

Press CV 12 and CV 6: Lie on your stomach and place the palm of your right hand over your solar plexus (CV 12), midway between the end of your breastbone and your belly button. If you have a serious illness such as heart disease, cancer, or high blood pressure or are on medication, consult your doctor first

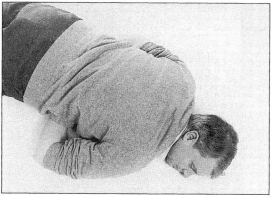

before doing this exercise. Place the palm of your left hand on CV 6 in between your pubic bone and belly button. Turn your head on its side, close your eyes, and begin long, deep breathing. You will probably feel some abdominal pain at the end of your exhalation.

---

[43] Practicing this routine on the floor provides a lot more pressure than does lying on your bed. If you find that your points are sore, practice on your bed; if you find you want more pressure, practice on a carpeted floor.

The pain usually begins to subside within five minutes. Train yourself to focus on breathing deeply instead of focusing on the pain. If you get tired easily or often feel weak, then limit the time you practice this exercise to one minute. After a week, you can gradually extend the time. Keep it up; perseverance pays off.

After the pain subsides, turn over and lie comfortably on your back.

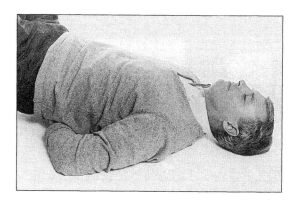

Step 2

Press B 23 and B 47: Lie on your back with your legs bent, feet flat on the floor. Raise your pelvis, placing your fists underneath your lower back. Position your knuckles between your spine and the thick, ropy muscles of your lower back. This will press both the inner (B 23) and outer (B 47) points. Relax your body down onto your fists, close your eyes, and breathe deeply into your stomach for one minute.

The rest of this routine can be practiced either sitting or lying down.

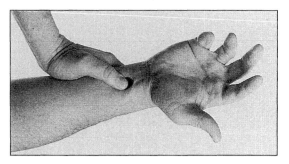

Step 3

Firmly press P 6: Place your left thumb on the inside of your right wrist, two-and-one-half finger widths below the center of the wrist crease. Pressing firmly with your thumb, place your fingertips directly behind, on the outside of your forearm. This point helps to settle the stomach and relieve nausea. Hold for one minute as you breathe deeply. Then switch sides to press the point on your other arm.

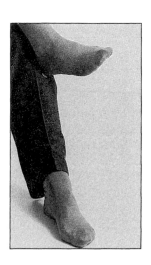

Step 4

Briskly rub St 36: With your left leg straight out , place your right heel on the left St 36 point. Briskly rub the point for thirty seconds using friction to create heat. Then do the same on the other leg to help strengthen and stabilize the digestive system.

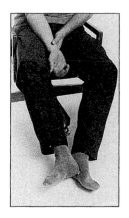

Step 5

Press Sp 4 with your opposite heel: With the outer edge of your left foot on the ground, place your right heel in the arch of your left foot to press Sp 4. Optional: While the heel presses Sp 4 in the arch of the foot, place your left thumb on the inside of your right forearm to press P 6 on your right side. Hold this point combination for one minute, breathing deeply. Then switch sides and hold these points for another minute.

Breathing deeply into your stomach is important for increasing the effectiveness of this routine. With each inhalation your belly should swell. With each exhalation, simply let your whole body relax.

For Abdominal Pain Due to Gas: Lie down on your back and simply bring your knees up to your chest. Hug your knees and breathe deeply for one minute. Then lie down comfortably with your legs bent, feet on the floor, and your eyes closed. Breathe deeply into your belly for two more minutes.

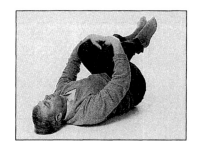

Additional Points for Relieving Stomachaches, Indigestion, and Heartburn

For illustrations of other related points for relieving stomachaches, indigestion, and heartburn, see chapter 12, "Constipation"; chapter 15, "Diarrhea"; and chapter 32, "Motion Sickness, Morning Sickness, and Nausea."

40
SWELLING AND WATER RETENTION

$\mathcal{A}$cupressure's potent points can relieve the discomforts caused by excessive water retention. In traditional Chinese medicine, edema (swelling due to water retention) is usually associated with weakness in the spleen and kidney meridians. By using the points along these meridians, acupressure restores the proper level of water for your system, tones muscles and tissues, and improves the body's fluid balance.

If swelling persists or is accompanied by headaches, fevers, severe pain, nausea, or skin disorders, always see your doctor to determine if there is an underlying condition that requires medical treatment.

When you maintain the same position — standing, for example — for a long period of time, the lack of movement and the constant weight on your feet inhibits blood circulation and causes swelling. Tight-fitting shoes can also lead to swollen feet and ankles.

Many overweight people retain water easily. Often, dieters cut their food consumption, but have difficulty losing their water weight. The acupressure points in this chapter facilitate weight loss by stimulating the metabolism to help the body shed excess water. When practiced regularly with relaxation and deep breathing exercises, these points also curb the appetite — an additional benefit to dieters.

Many women suffer from premenstrual bloating, which contributes to irritability and emotional distress. Practicing these points along with deep breathing and relaxation exercises regularly before and during your period can relieve and prevent this condition. These same points not only relieve bloating and the symptoms of PMS, they also regulate menstruation.

A low-sodium diet is recommended for preventing swelling, because excess salt causes the body to retain water.

The following acupressure points relieve as well as prevent swollen feet and ankles, premenstrual bloating, facial puffiness due to congestion, and other swelling caused by water retention.

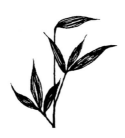

Potent Points for Relieving Swelling and Water Retention

Sea of Energy (CV 6)

Location: Two finger widths directly below the belly button.

Benefits: Relieves water retention, chronic diarrhea, constipation, and gas.

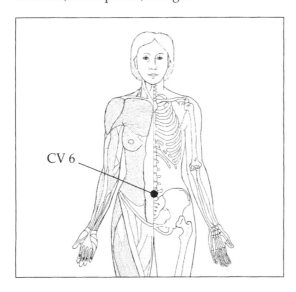

Shady Side of the Mountain (Sp 9)

Location: On the inside of the leg below the knee and under the large bulge of the bone.

Benefits: Relieves knee problems, swelling, leg tension, varicose veins, edema, water retention, and cramps.

Three Yin Crossing (Sp 6)

Caution: Do not stimulate this point during the eighth and ninth months of pregnancy.

Location: Four finger widths above the inner anklebone on the back inner border of the shinbone.

Benefits: Relieves water retention and edema; a special trigger point for vaginal complaints and swelling.

Blazing Valley (K 2)

Location: On the middle of the arch of the foot midway between the outer tip of the big toe and the back of the heel.

Benefits: Relieves edema, especially swollen feet.

Illuminated Sea (K 6)

Location: One thumb width below the inside of the anklebone.

Benefits: Relieves water retention, especially swollen ankles.

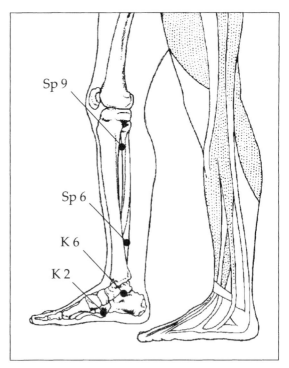

■ *You do not have to use all of these points. Using just one or two of them can be effective.*

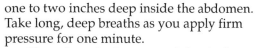

Potent Point Exercises

Although you can practice this routine sitting, it is most effective when done lying down on your back, with your knees bent and your feet flat on the floor.

Step 1

Firmly press CV 6: Place all of your fingertips of both hands between the pubic bone and belly button in your lower abdominal area. Take long, deep breaths as you gradually press one to two inches deep inside the abdomen. Take long, deep breaths as you apply firm pressure for one minute.

If you have had a recent abdominal operation or have a serious, life-threatening illness (see caution on page 9) such as heart disease, cancer, or high blood pressure, consult your doctor before you press this abdominal point. Light, gentle pressure may be appropriate to your condition.

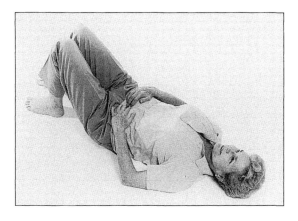

Step 2

Lightly press Sp 9 with Sp 6: With your legs bent and your feet flat on the floor, place your right foot comfortably on your left thigh. Use your right thumb to press the right Sp 9 point in the indentation in the bone (tibia) below the inside of your knee. Angle the pressure underneath the bone, up toward the knee. This point is often tender, so press gently. Use your left thumb to press into a slight indentation in the inner border of your shinbone, four finger widths above the inner anklebone. Close your eyes as you hold these two potent points and breathe deeply for one minute. End by holding these points lightly as you take two more long, deep breaths. Then switch legs to hold these points on the other side for another minute. If one of your legs is more swollen than the other, gently hold the more swollen side twice as long.

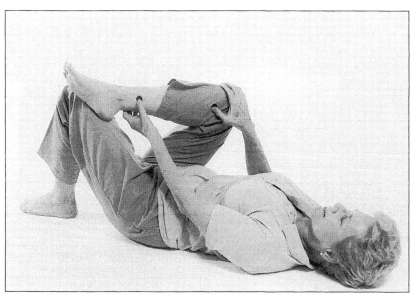

Step 3

Press K 2 and K 6: Once again, place your right foot on the top of your left thigh. Use your right fingertips to press K 6 on your right foot, in the indentation between your inner anklebone and your heel. Feel for a thin, wiry band or a sore spot. Place your left thumb on the center of the arch of your right foot. Angle your finger pressure up and underneath the bone structure, with the other fingers on the top of the foot. Hold these points for one minute. Then switch legs and continue to breathe deeply.

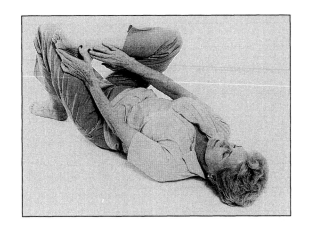

Additional Points for Relieving Swelling and Water Retention

For illustrations of other related points for relieving swelling and water retention, see chapter 5, "Ankle and Foot Problems"; chapter 31, "Menstrual Tension, Cramps, and PMS"; and chapter 38, "Sinus Problems and Hay Fever."

41

TOOTHACHES

*T*ooth pain can be caused by tooth decay or an injury that exposes the nerves in the root canal. Toothaches as well as the pain associated with gum disease can be temporarily relieved by applying acupressure. However, it is still necessary to see your dentist to treat the cause of the toothache.

Traditionally, the acupressure points on the large intestine meridian have been used for relieving toothaches. This channel travels from the hands, up the arms, and into the gums and teeth. This is why trigger points in these areas can help tooth pain.

Avoid eating cold foods and especially foods that contain sugar. To relieve the pain of a toothache, you can also rub oil of cloves onto the surrounding gums.

I have used self-acupressure effectively while in my dentist's office, during drilling to fill a cavity. Deep pressure on the LI 4 point between the thumb and index finger numbs most of the pain without using any novocaine.

Special Arm Points

A series of acupressure points on the outside of the upper arm can also relieve toothaches. If the affected tooth is on the right side of your mouth, then use the points on your right arm; if it is in a back molar, then find the tender spots in the back of your upper, outer arm. If the toothache is toward the front of your mouth, look for a sore point on the front of your upper arm.

Curve your fingers, using your fingertips to hold directly and firmly on the sorest point

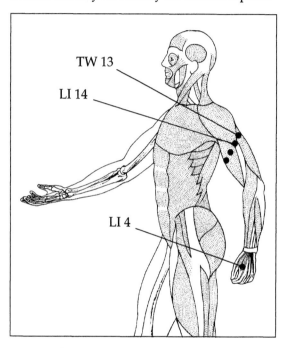

you can find on the outside of your upper arm. Hold for several minutes, until the arm soreness and the toothache both subside. This can be a good technique to teach your children to give them a sense of self-control and counteract fear and helplessness when going to the dentist. Children can learn to control their pain, too, and choose new ways of concentrating.

Potent Points for Relieving Toothaches

Jaw Chariot (St 6)

Location: Between the upper and lower jaws, on the muscle in front of the earlobe that bulges when the back teeth are slightly clenched.

Benefits: Relieves jaw pain and spasm, TMJ problems, lockjaw, sore throats, dental neuralgia, and toothaches.

Facial Beauty (St 3)

Location: At the bottom of the cheekbone, directly below the pupil.

Benefits: Relieves toothaches, head congestion, and sinus pain.

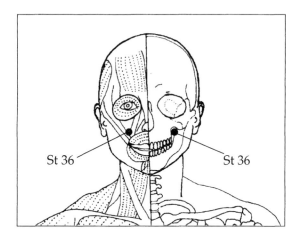

Joining the Valley (Hoku) (LI 4)

Caution: This point is forbidden for pregnant women because its stimulation can cause premature contractions in the uterus.

Location: In the webbing between the thumb and index finger at the highest spot of the muscle when the thumb and index finger are brought close together.

Benefits: Relieves headaches and toothaches; also traditionally used as a general pain reliever, decongestant, and anti-inflammatory point.

Shoulder Meeting Point (TW 13)

Location: On the outer surface of the upper arm, one thumb width in back of the base of the upper arm muscle (the deltoid) and two finger widths higher up toward the shoulder.

Benefits: Relieves toothaches, elbow pain, shoulder pain, and painful arm extension.

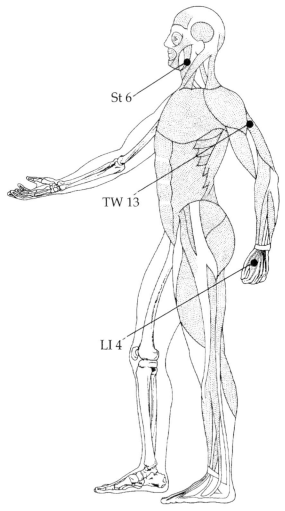

■ *You do not have to use all of these points. Using just one or two of them whenever you have a free hand can be effective.*

Potent Point Exercises

Sit comfortably to stimulate the following points on the same side of the body on which you have the toothache. For best results, use firm enough pressure to trigger tolerable pain or tenderness.

Step 1

Firmly press St 6 along with St 3: Place your thumbs between the upper and lower jaws, to press St 6 firmly on the jaw muscle. With your fingers curved, place your index and middle fingertips beside your nose and press up underneath your cheekbones. Close your eyes and take long, deep breaths as you continue to press these toothache relief points for one minute.

Step 2

Hold LI 4 and TW 13: Press these toothache relief trigger points on the same side that your toothache is on. First, stimulate LI 4 in the webbing between the thumb and index finger for one minute. Then press TW 13 on the outside of your upper arm. Rub your fingers over the outside of the arm to feel for a sore spot. Press right on the most tender area for two minutes, and breathe deeply until the pain or tenderness subsides.

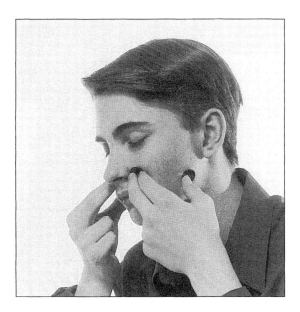

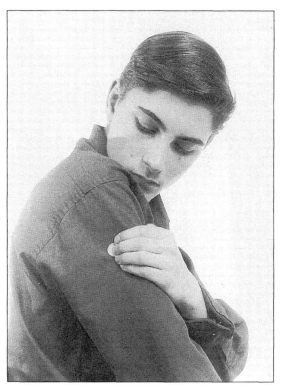

Additional Points for Relieving Toothaches

For illustrations of other related points for relieving toothache, see chapter 20, "Headaches and Migraines"; and chapter 27, "Jaw Problems (TMJ Problems)."

42

WRIST PAIN

(CARPAL TUNNEL SYNDROME AND TENDONITIS)

I once met a renowned baseball player after a twilight double-header. He was holding his right wrist in pain. After I applied deep finger pressure on his wrist, arm, and shoulders he told me that he had been worried that his wrist pain would keep him from finishing the season — but the pain was now gone, and he felt confident he could continue.

Few joints in the body are as as important for carrying out daily activities as the joints in the hands and wrists. When aches or pains occur in the wrist joint, it is useful to know natural ways to help yourself. As a hands-on health care therapy, acupressure has been found effective for relieving many types of hand pain, from a sprained wrist to carpal tunnel syndrome and wrist tendonitis. Dr. Keith Kenyon also found that acupressure relieved wrist arthritis.[44]

Carpal Tunnel Syndrome results from swelling that creates pressure on the medial nerve. Tendonitis is an inflammation of the tendons due to overuse. Daily acupressure on the potent points in this chapter can relieve wrist pain and inflammation as well as promote healing.

The following acupressure points and methods can relax the tendons and muscles that attach to the wrist, allowing greater use of the fingers with less pain and discomfort. I have discovered that making gentle hand movements, such as rotating the hand, while pressing the points around the wrist with the knuckles of the other hand often increases the effectiveness of the acupressure.[45]

---

[44] Keith Kenyon, M.D., *Do-It-Yourself Acupuncture Without Needles* (New York: Arco Publishing, 1977), 71.
[45] Refer to Michael Reed Gach, *Arthritis Relief at Your Fingertips* (London: Piatkus Books, 1989), 71-74, 88-90.

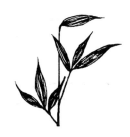

Potent Points for Relieving Wrist Pain

Inner Gate (P 6)

Location: In the middle of the inner side of the forearm, two and one-half finger widths below the wrist crease.

Benefits: Relieves nausea, anxiety, and wrist pain.

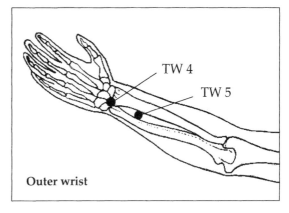

Outer wrist

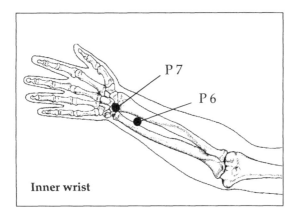

Inner wrist

Big Mound (P 7)

Location: In the middle of the inside of the wrist crease.

Benefits: Relieves wrist problems, such as carpal tunnel syndrome, rheumatism, and wrist tendonitis.

■ *You do not have to use all of these points. Using just one or two of them whenever you have a free hand can be effective.*

Outer Gate (TW 5)

Location: On the outside of the forearm, midway between the two bones (radius and ulna), two and one-half finger widths below the wrist crease.

Benefits: Relieves rheumatism, tendonitis, and wrist pain; increases resistance to colds.

Active Pond (TW 4)

Location: Follow the outside of the arm to the hollow in the center of the wrist at the crease.

Benefits: Relieves wrist tendonitis, rheumatism, pain when grasping, carpal tunnel syndrome, and wrist pain; also strengthens the wrist.

Potent Point Exercises

This short routine is designed to be practiced while sitting comfortably.

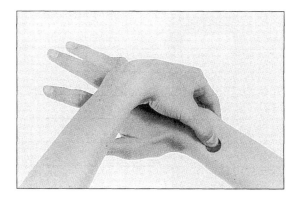

Step 1:

Firmly press TW 5 and P 6: Place the fingers of your left hand on top of your right forearm and your thumb directly behind your fingers on the other side, two and one-half finger widths below the wrist crease. Grasp these points firmly for one minute to strengthen the wrist joint. Then switch sides to work on your left wrist for another minute. If grasping hurts your hand, use your knuckles on these points instead.

Step 2:

Hold P 7 and TW 4: Place your left thumb on the center of the outer wrist crease, with your fingers directly behind on the inside of the wrist. Fit your thumb and fingers, as shown, or use your knuckles in the hollow spaces between the bones. Gradually apply firm pressure and begin long, deep breathing. Press these points for one minute or until you feel your wrist pain subside. End by holding lightly, taking another couple of long, slow, deep breaths. Feel for a pulsation at the point. Then switch sides to work on your opposite wrist for another minute.

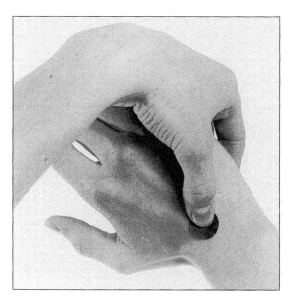

Most importantly — for any wrist injury elevate your hand to decrease the swelling!

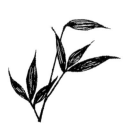

43

ACUPRESSURE WELLNESS PROGRAM

*T*he choices we make in our lives, how we think, use our bodies, eat, sleep, exercise, and set our priorities, affect our health and wellness. The more conscious we are of giving our bodies what they require, the more we take responsibility for our well-being. Preventing illness is just as important as healing illness, and yet many people don't become concerned with their health until they get sick.

The Acupressure Wellness Program is a holistic approach to health maintenance that combines daily self-acupressure with choices for a healthy lifestyle, including good nutrition, exercise, positive thinking, relaxation, and deep breathing.

Acupressure and Deep Breathing for Health Maintenance

The acupressure points illustrated in this book not only relieve common ailments, they are also effective for preventing them. I recommend regular use of the acupressure tonic points in chapter 23, "Immune System Boosting," to strengthen the whole body. By stimulating these points daily, you can improve your overall condition and also increase your vitality.

Deep breathing exercises are the most gentle and effective methods known for purifying and revitalizing the body. If your breathing is shallow, your body's vital systems are not functioning at their optimal levels. When you breathe deeply, however, the

respiratory system can fully oxygenate and rejuvenate the body.

Daily Exercise

Stretching and aerobic exercise are the two most important types of exercise to practice daily for health maintenance. Gentle stretching (five minutes, twice a day) keeps your muscles and joints loose. Aerobic exercise (twenty to thirty minutes a day) — swimming, bicycling, running, or brisk walking — develops muscle tone, stimulates deep breathing and sweating, and increases blood circulation.

Exercise naturally regulates and balances your whole system. When you don't exercise, your metabolism can become sluggish and the tendency to get depressed or to overeat increases. When you exercise regularly, though, you tend to develop a healthy appetite, a positive frame of mind, and an overall increase in vitality.

Diet

Diet also plays an important role in health maintenance and resistance to illness. When we eat processed, preserved, or devitalized foods, we weaken our system. However, there are foods that strengthen the body and build resistance, reinforcing the body's ability to protect itself. The following chart summarizes the best foods to eat, which to eat in moderation, and which to avoid.

Healthy Foods

Vegetables
Whole grains
Seeds (in moderation)
Nuts (in moderation)
Beans (in moderation)
Tofu and miso soup
Fish and seaweed
Fresh fruits

Foods to Avoid

Processed foods with sugar
White flour products
Salt (eat less)
Fried foods (eat less)
Dairy products (eat less)
Red meat
Chemical additives
Coffee, including decaffeinated (drink less)

The Five-Minute Acupressure Wellness Exercise

I would like to leave you with this short potent point routine to maintain your health and relieve stress. It can easily be practiced at home or at work. Begin by sitting forward on the front edge of a straight-backed chair.

Step 1

Briskly rub your lower back. Do not press on disintegrating discs or on fractured or broken bones. If your lower back is tender, use a light touch. Otherwise, place the backs of your hands against your lower back along both sides of the spine. Rub these Sea of Vitality points (B 23 and B 47) briskly up and down for one minute, creating warmth from the friction.

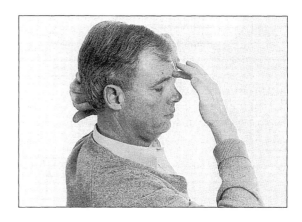

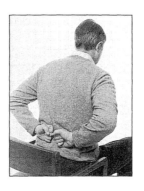

Step 2

Hold the base of the skull with the Third Eye point. Tilt your head back, close your eyes, and practice the following deep breathing meditation.

Take three long, slow, deep breaths. Imagine that each deep breath brings a healing substance that penetrates and dissolves your pain or tension. Concentrate on breathing deeply into any stress or tight muscles. Hold each breath for a couple of seconds at the top of the inhalation. Exhale, smoothly letting go of your tension. Continue breathing deeply for one more minute, visualizing each breath carrying healing energy into your body.

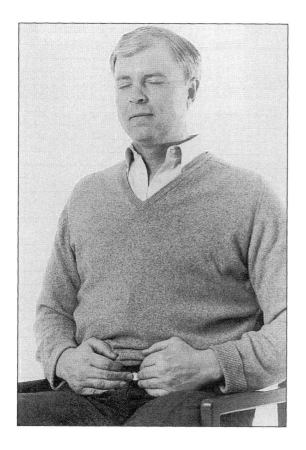

Step 3

Hold the Sea of Energy (CV 6) three fingers width below your belly button in your lower abdomen.

Now sit back comfortably in your chair with your spine straight and your shoulders relaxed. Close your eyes, press firmly into this potent point, and breathe deeply for one minute.

Everyone can be radiantly healthy by eating wholesome foods, thinking positively, practicing stretching and deep breathing exercises, and getting daily aerobic exercise.

Press your potent points whenever you have a free hand and you will enjoy greater aliveness, vitality, and well-being.

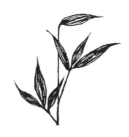

APPENDIX A:
POINT LOCATION CHARTS

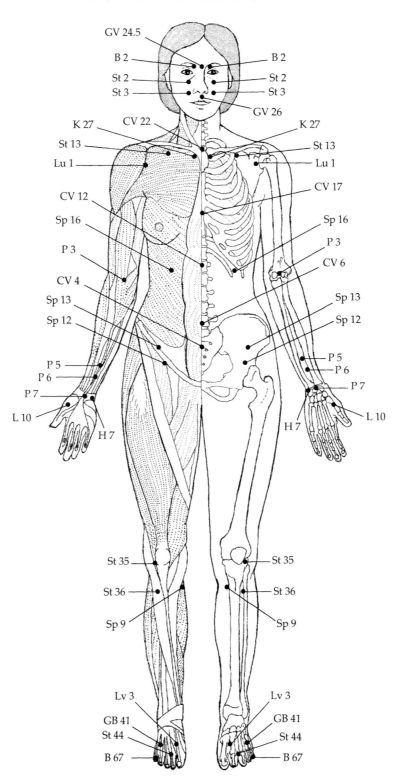

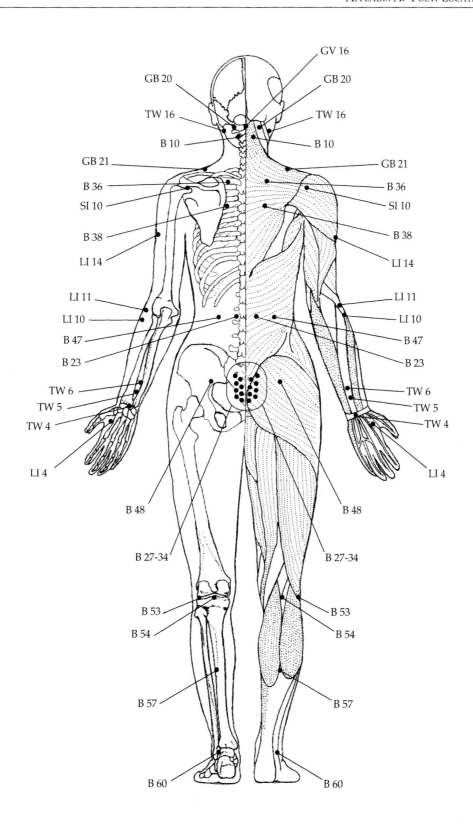

GV 16

GB 20　　　　　　　　　　　　　　　　GB 20

TW 16　　　　　　　　　　　　　　　　TW 16

B 10　　　　　　　　　　　　　　　　B 10

GB 21　　　　　　　　　　　　　　　　GB 21

B 36　　　　　　　　　　　　　　　　B 36

SI 10　　　　　　　　　　　　　　　　SI 10

B 38　　　　　　　　　　　　　　　　B 38

LI 14　　　　　　　　　　　　　　　　LI 14

LI 11　　　　　　　　　　　　　　　　LI 11

LI 10　　　　　　　　　　　　　　　　LI 10

B 47　　　　　　　　　　　　　　　　B 47

B 23　　　　　　　　　　　　　　　　B 23

TW 6　　　　　　　　　　　　　　　　TW 6

TW 5　　　　　　　　　　　　　　　　TW 5

TW 4　　　　　　　　　　　　　　　　TW 4

LI 4　　　　　　　　　　　　　　　　LI 4

B 48　　　　　　　　　　　　　　　　B 48

B 27-34　　　　　　　　　　　　　　　　B 27-34

B 53　　　　　　　　　　　　　　　　B 53

B 54　　　　　　　　　　　　　　　　B 54

B 57　　　　　　　　　　　　　　　　B 57

B 60　　　　　　　　　　　　　　　　B 60

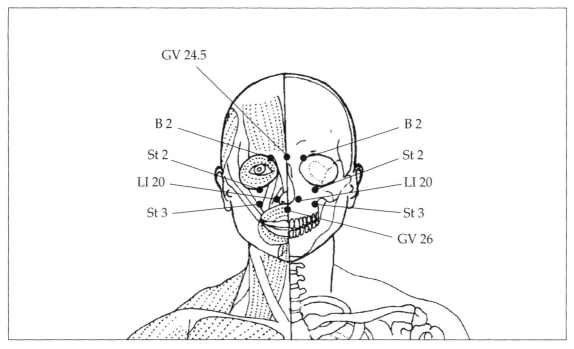

GV 24.5

B 2   B 2

St 2   St 2

LI 20   LI 20

St 3   St 3

GV 26

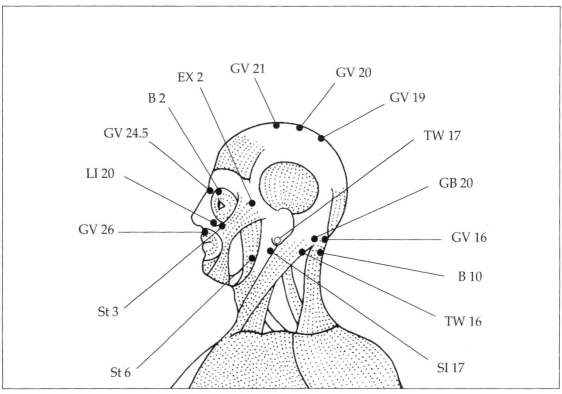

EX 2   GV 21   GV 20

B 2   GV 19

GV 24.5   TW 17

LI 20   GB 20

GV 26   GV 16

                      B 10

St 3   TW 16

St 6   SI 17

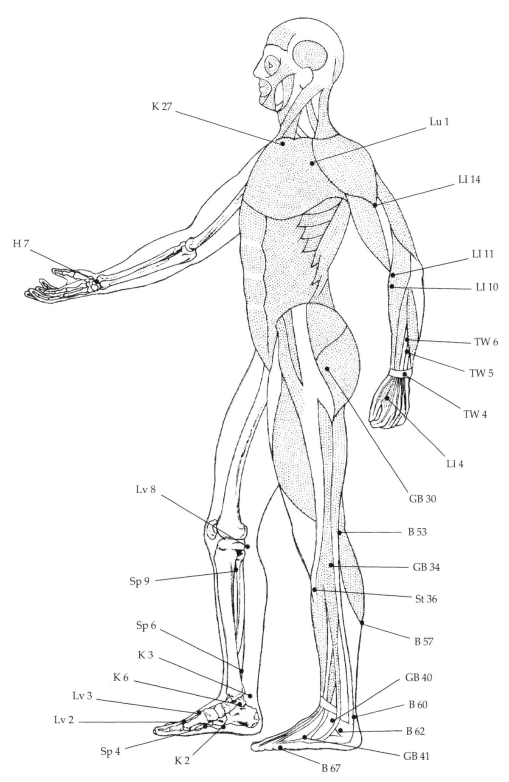

K 27

Lu 1

LI 14

H 7

LI 11

LI 10

TW 6

TW 5

TW 4

LI 4

GB 30

Lv 8

B 53

GB 34

Sp 9

St 36

Sp 6

B 57

K 3

K 6

GB 40

Lv 3

B 60

Lv 2

B 62

Sp 4

GB 41

K 2

B 67

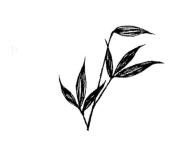

Potent Points Summary

POTENT POINTS	PAGE NUMBERS

Abdominal Sorrow Sp 16
Relieves indigestion, nausea, and abdominal cramps; balances   82, 99, 110, 174
appetite and the gastrointestinal system

Above Tears GB 41
Relieves headaches, sideaches, sciatica, and arthritic pains;   105
reduces water retention

Active Pond TW 4
Relieves wrist tendonitis and rheumatism; moistens dryness   222
and relieves wrist pain

Anterior Summit GV 21
Aids psychological conflicts, trauma, and headaches; clears the   77
brain; calms the spirit

Big Mound P 7
Relieves wrist problems and emotional imbalances; benefits the   222
wrist and regulates the stomach

Bigger Rushing Lv 3
Relieves arthritis cramps, headaches, tired eyes, and hangovers;   26, 55, 73, 90, 99, 105, 120,
alleviates congestion and pain; invigorates, transforms, and   155, 163
clears the system

Bigger Stream K 3
Relieves difficult labor, fatigue, swollen feet, and insomnia;   32, 86, 120, 127, 152, 188
restores the immune and reproductive systems

Blazing Valley K 2
Relieves irregular menstruation, swelling, and foot cramps;   214
benefits the kidneys and relieves swollen feet

Breast Root St 18
Relieves breast pains, lactation problems, chest pain, and   158
heartburn; governs the breast and calms the spirit

POTENT POINTS	PAGE NUMBERS

POTENT POINTS   PAGE NUMBERS

Drilling Bamboo B 2
Relieves sinus pain, headaches, foggy vision, and hay fever; 60, 90, 99, 104, 178, 202
clears the sinuses and brightens the eyes

Ear Gate TW 21
Relieves ear pain or soreness and hearing and TMJ problems; 86, 144
opens and benefits the ears

Elegant Mansion K 27
Relieves anxiety, hiccups, coughing, and sore throats; benefits 27, 44, 61, 64, 78, 111, 119
the lungs, throat, and kidneys

Eyes Bright B 1
Relieves severe nosebleeds; alleviates eye pain 182

Facial Beauty St 3
Relieves head congestion, stuffy nose, and burning eyes; clears 21, 60, 90, 99, 105, 182, 202,
the sinuses and the face 218

Fish Border Lu 10
Relieves breathing difficulties, asthma, and emotional distress; 44
clears the lungs and relieves wrist pain.

Four Whites St 2
Relieves acne, facial blemishes, and burning eyes; clears and 21, 90, 127, 169
relaxes the eyes and face

Gate Origin CV 4
Relieves impotency, urinary incontinence, and insomnia; 127
strengthens the reproductive system

Gates of Consciousness GB 20
Relieves stiff necks, headaches, insomnia, and hypertension; 54, 60, 98, 104, 114, 133,
alleviates head and neck pain 140, 144, 162, 186, 188, 198

Grandfather Grandson Sp 4
Relieves abdominal and menstrual cramps, stomachaches, 82, 169, 210
indigestion, and anxiety; regulates and strengthens digestion

Great Abyss Lu 9
Relieves asthma, coughing, irritability, and agitation; balances 44
the lungs

POTENT POINTS	PAGE NUMBERS

POTENT POINTS	PAGE NUMBERS
Jumping Circle GB 30 Relieves frustration, irritation, hip pain, and rheumatism; relaxes the tendons and restores joint mobility	139
Letting Go Lu 1 Relieves difficult breathing, asthma, fatigue, confusion, and irritability; clears the chest and emotions and strengthens the lungs	44, 54, 78, 111, 139, 158
Listening Place SI 19 Relieves earaches, water in the ear, ear pressure, and TMJ problems and balances the thyroid gland	86, 144
Lung Associated B 13 Relieves breathing difficulties, chest	44
Mansion Cottage Sp 13 Relieves impotency, menstrual cramps, and abdominal discomfort; relieves abdominal pain, bloating, and cramps	127, 168, 193
Middle of a Person GV 26 Relieves cramps, fainting, dizziness, and hay fever; revives the consciousness, relieves pain, and clears the brain	73, 162, 182, 203
One Hundred Meeting Point GV 20 Relieves hot flashes, heatstroke headaches, and epilepsy; clears the brain and calms the spirit; good for memory and concentration	77, 115, 162, 202
Outer Arm Bone LI 14 Relieves aching in the arms, shoulder tension, stiff necks, and toothaches; relaxes the shoulder muscles	198
Outer Gate TW 5 Relieves allergic reactions, rheumatism, and tendonitis; regulates and relaxes the entire body	26, 55, 120, 222
Penetrate Heaven B 7 Relieves headaches, and nasal and head congestion; clears the nose	202
Posterior Summit GV 19 Aids psychological conflicts, trauma, and headaches; clears the brain, and calms the spirit	77

POTENT POINTS	PAGE NUMBERS
Spirit Gate H 7 Relieves insomnia due to overexcitement and relieves anxiety; regulates the heart and strengthens the spirit	36, 133
Sun Point CV 22 Counteracts poor memory; relieves cold with a headache and eye pain; strengthens the brain, and brightens the eyes	162
Sunny Side of the Mountain GB 34 Relieves knee pain, sciatica, and muscular problems; relaxes the muscles of the lower body	148
Supporting Mountain B 57 Relieves cramps, stomachaches, leg pain and swelling; relaxes the calf muscle and strengthens the lower back	73
Third Eye Point GV 24.5 Relieves glandular imbalances, irritability, depression, and confusion; stimulates immune functioning and calms the spirit	21, 36, 55, 61, 78, 90, 99, 104, 114, 115, 133, 140, 158, 163, 186, 193, 203
Three Mile Point St 36 Relieves fatigue, stomach disorders, and nausea; benefits digestion and restores the immune system	20, 27, 55, 68, 78, 82, 119, 127, 148, 155, 163, 174, 188, 210
Three Yin Crossing Sp 6 Relieves water retention, diarrhea, menstrual cramps, and diabetes; regulates menstruation and balances the uroreproductive system	169, 214
Travel Between Lv 2 Relieves diarrhea, stomachaches, and nausea; calms the spirit	82
Vital Diaphragm B 38 Relieves breathing difficulties, anxiety, and hypertension; calms the emotions and promotes relaxation	63
Welcoming Perfume LI 20 Relieves stuffy nose, sinus pain, and nasal congestion; clears the nose and sinuses	60, 202
Wilderness Mound GB 40 Relieves ankle sprains, sciatic pain, sideaches, shoulder pain, and headaches	32

GLOSSARY

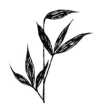

Acupressure: An ancient healing art that uses finger pressure on the acupuncture points and meridians to release muscular pain and tensions, and to increase circulation.

Acupuncture: Inserts fine needles into the body at points and meridians to relieve pain and treat various ailments.

Acu-Yoga: Uses full-body postures to stretch the meridians and stimulate the acupressure points along with deep breathing.

Affirmations: Positive statements that acknowledge life, said aloud or silently. Affirmations reinforce the power of positive thinking and can be used to enhance the benefits of acupressure.

Arthritis: Joint inflammation that causes pain and often limits the range of motion.

Blockage: Congestion of an area of the body that may ache, be tense, or feel numb.

Breath Visualization: Using the power of concentration to direct long, deep breaths into specific areas of the body.

Centering: Gaining awareness of the body in the present moment.

Chi: The Chinese term for the energy that circulates through pathways called meridians.

Chronic Tension: A long-term contracted muscular condition.

Distal Points: Acupressure located a distance from the area they benefit. *See Local Points.*

Homeostasis: The state of equilibrium or balance.

Impotence: Lacking in physical strength and the inability to engage in sexual intercourse.

Lateral: Toward the outside of the body.

Life Force: The vital energy contained in all things that circulates through the meridians.

Local Points: Acupressure points located in the area they benefit. *See Distal Points.*

Lumbar Vertebrae: The last five bones on the lower back above the base of the spine.

Medial: Toward the center of the body.

Meditation: Focusing attention to develop the spiritual capabilities of the mind.

Meridian: Human energy pathways that connect the various acupressure and acupuncture points and the internal organs.

Standard Meridian Abbreviations	
Lu	Lung
LI	Large Intestine
Sp	Spleen
TW	Triple Warmer
St	Stomach
SI	Small Intestine
H	Heart
CV	Conception Vessel
K	Kidney
P	Pericardium
B	Bladder
GB	Gallbladder
Lv	Liver
GV	Governing Vessel
EX	Extra Point

Metatarsals: The bones between the ankle and toes, on the top of the foot.

Pressure Points: Places on the body along a meridian with high levels of electrical conductivity.

Referred Pain: Pain generated in one area of the body, but felt in another.

Sacrum: The flat triangular bone in the lower back at the base of the spine.

Sacroiliac Joints: The two places in the lower back where the sacrum joins the hipbones.

Shiatsu: A Japanese style of acupressure using firm finger pressure on points along the meridians.

Thoracic Vertebrae: The twelve spinal vertebrae below the neck in the upper and middle back.

Trigger Point: Same as an acupressure point; specific body locations that, when pressed with the fingers, relieve tension, pain, or pressure.

Index

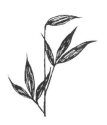

E

OTHER BOOKS BY MICHAEL REED GACH

Arthritis Relief at Your Fingertips (*Piatkus Books*)
Greater Energy at Your Fingertips (*Celestial Arts*)
Acu-Yoga: Self-help techniques to relieve tension (*Japan Publications*)
The Bum Back Book: Acupressure self-help back care (*Celestial Arts*)

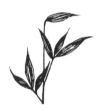

Audio and Videotapes

The Acupressure Institute in Berkeley, California sells a wide variety of educational materials, including acupressure books, charts, flash cards, and special instructional audio and videotapes on how to do acupressure. Michael Reed Gach has made tapes on the following:

Arthritis Relief Audiotapes
Tape 1 Morning and Evening Routines
Tape 2 Self-Acupressure Techniques
Tape 3 Self-Care for Relieving Hand Pain

Refresher Audiotapes
The 5:00 Refresher: Revitalize yourself after work
The Traveller's Refresher: You'll arrive feeling great!
The Smoker's Refresher: Extra energy to break the habit
The Rush Hour Refresher: Relieve stress while you drive
The Wake-up Refresher: A boost of energy to start the day
Greater Energy at Your Fingertips: Relieve stress and recharge

For Women Only Audiotapes
Weight Loss: Decrease hunger and fatigue
PMS Relief: Relieve menstrual discomfort or cramps
Greater Beauty: Enjoy a natural, non-surgical facelift
Techniques for Greater Energy: Revitalize yourself!

Acupressure Videotapes
The Bum Back Video
Releasing Shoulder and Neck Tension
Zen Shiatsu Instruction (for practitioners)
Fundamentals of Acupressure

Write to *The Acupressure Institute, 1533 Shattuck Avenue, Berkeley, California 94709, USA (800 442 2232)* to receive a free colour brochure and mail order form. Website: www.acupressureinstitute.com

Shiatsu is a form of acupressure popular in the UK. For more information, contact *The Shiatsu Society*, PO Box 4580, Rugby, Warwickshire CV21 9EL Website: www.shiatsusociety.org

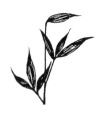